Nourishing Hope™
for Autism

Nutrition & Diet for Healing Our Children

Julie Matthews
Certified Nutrition Consultant

3ⁿᵈ Edition: Revised September 2008

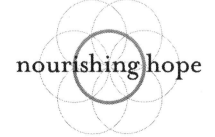

nourishing hope

Acknowledgements

I have been working on this book in one way or another for seven years. Every step of the way, information and people I needed seemed to unfold before me. In my opinion, a true sign of what was meant to be.

The angel I'm most grateful for is Anita Kugelstadt, my editor, and the mom of a child with autism who offered me her editing services with nothing expected in return—simply the desire to help other parents by helping me get this work out there. Anita made sure that the book was readable. She lent a critical eye that could ensure it was scientifically sound and referenced for accuracy for professionals interested in the science. But most importantly she shared her experience as a parent—on this path for a while—who was able to remember her first experience with all of this information, enabling me to provide clear answers to the questions asked by parents new to biomedical. She also ensured that I included information for "non-responders" and more complex situations, so that this book could help parents anywhere along the road —new parents, children that responded quickly to simply interventions, and nuances for those who have been working with diet for years. Anita's perspective, knowledge, and hard work were helpful beyond words.

This heart and spirit of Anita, I see reflected in many. And I am so grateful for everyone who offered assistance. Trudy Scott, CN (Certified Nutritionist), my research assistant, spent many days helping gather crucial scientific references. Her knowledge of nutrition, project management ability and interest in the subject, were essential. She worked long, hard hours pulling the final pieces of this book together, and again, she asked for nothing in return. I could not have done it without her.

There were also several wonderful women who lent their passion and knowledge out of the kindness of their hearts. Kelli Pallett, who initially offered to edit for me, then later invited me to speak to parents in Toronto. Unknown friends responded to my email, offering to help me as I pulled together many more pieces of research. I genuinely appreciate their efforts. Thank you Marjie, Bonnie, Wendy, Cynthia, Kerry, and Nicole.

All of these women have demonstrated what I love so much about the autism community—we are a family. We are all on the same team. We are here to support each other. The love, commitment, and strength of these mothers, fathers, and professionals are so powerful that I am often brought to tears. This is a labor of love for me.

I thank all of the parents—known and unknown. You provide me strength in my own life to face the trials and tribulations that affect us all as humans through your unending hope, faith, and perseverance. Your knowledge is often greater than mine—I am humbled by it, and I learn so much from you all.

Thank you to all the clinicians and scientists who have stood up for the truth—often at great risk to their own livelihood. You are true heroes.

Finally, to my husband, my greatest support, who believes in me more than I believe in myself at times. You have supported me physically and emotionally when the pressure felt too much. You encouraged me to follow my passion and do what I felt was right - regardless of what others said I "should" do. Your unconditional love has allowed me to become my complete self. With you by my side, I can create freely and share openly.

Though I do not have a child on the autism spectrum, I was drawn to help from the first day I learned the biochemistry of autism. Something in my heart told me this was right and I became driven to share so that others may benefit from applying nutrition and diet toward healing and wellness. My passion to continue learning stems from my commitment to seek answers and identify solutions.

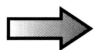

Biochemical Imbalances **Neurological Disorder**

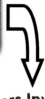

HOLISTIC NUTRITION APPROACH

1) Cleaning up The Diet
2) Cleaning up The Home
3) Supplement Basics
4) Diet Basics
5) Choosing a Foundational ASD Diet
6) Addressing Food Intolerances
7) Evolving the Diet:
8) Refining the ASD Diet
9) Cleaning up The Gut
10) Supplement Specifics
11) Support Immune Function
12) Detoxification

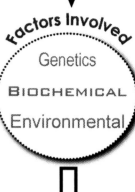

Factors Involved

Genetics
BIOCHEMICAL
Environmental

Nourishing Hope for Autism

Contents at a Glance

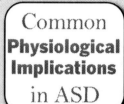

Common **Physiological Implications** in ASD

Liver & Detoxification

Immune System & Inflammation

GI Tract & Digestion

Endocrine & Glandular Function

Tying it all Back to The Brain

Gluten-Free Casein Free (GFCF)

Specific Carbohydrate Diet (SCD)

Weston A. Price Diet

Low Oxalate Diet

Raw Food Diet

Food Sensitivities

Feingold/Phenol

Body Ecology Diet

Paleolithic Diet

Feast Without Yeast

GAPS Diet

ASD Diet Options

Vitamins

Minerals

Amino Acids

Essential Fatty Acids

GI Supplements

Additional Supplements

IMPACT of Nutrients

NUTRITIONAL STRATEGIES & OPPORTUNITY

Contents

HOW TO READ THIS BOOK 1

PREFACE 3

INTRODUCTION 5

    BIOCHEMICAL IMBALANCES CREATE A NEUROLOGICAL DISORDER 5

PART ONE - GENETICS, ENVIRONMENTAL, AND BIOCHEMICAL FACTORS 7

    THE ETIOLOGY OF AUTISM: GENETICS AND ENVIRONMENTAL 9

    TOXINS CAN ALTER GENETICS 10

    ENVIRONMENT AND BIOCHEMISTRY: EFFECTS UPON EACH OTHER 11

GENETICS 13

    G-ALPHA PROTEIN DEFECT 14

    POLYMORPHISMS ASSOCIATED WITH METHYLATION 14

    OTHER POLYMORPHISMS 15

    EPIGENETICS AND DNA METHYLATION 15

    FAMILY HISTORY AND COMMON DISORDERS 16

ENVIRONMENTAL FACTORS AND BIOCHEMICAL IMPACT 19

    MERCURY TOXICITY 19

        Types of Mercury *19*

        Effects of Mercury *20*

        Mercury in Autism *20*

        Sources of Exposure *22*

            Amalgams 22

            Diet 23

            Air 24

            Vaccines and what they used to contain 24

            Vaccines and what they contain now, including synergistic impact 25

    OTHER HEAVY METALS 26

    ENVIRONMENTAL TOXINS 27

    VACCINATIONS AND IMMUNE FUNCTION 27

        MMR (Measles, Mumps, Rubella) Vaccination *29*

        Measles *29*

        Congenital Rubella *31*

        DTP (Diphtheria, Tetanus, and Pertussis) Vaccination *31*

    CANDIDA OVERGROWTH 32

    EAR INFECTIONS/ANTIBIOTICS 34

    FOOD SENSITIVITIES 34

    METHYLATION, TRANSSULFURATION, AND SULFATION 36

        Transsulfuration *43*

            Glutathione 43

            Metallothioneins 44

        Sulfation *44*

            Basics and Background on Sulfate and Sulfation 44

            Sulfation Function: Research and Clinical Observation 45

            Causes of Faulty Sulfation 46

            Sulfation and Phenols 47

        Sulfate and Sulfation in Systems Impaired in Autism *48*

        Sulfate and Detoxification *48*

        Sulfate in Gut and Brain Permeability *49*

        Sulfate and Digestion *50*

        Sulfate and Neurodevelopment *52*

        Sulfate and Immune Function *53*

COMMON PHYSIOLOGICAL IMPLICATIONS IN ASD **54**

    LIVER AND DETOXIFICATION 54
        Liver function *54*
        Detoxification in Autism *54*
    IMMUNE SYSTEM AND INFLAMMATION 54
        Immune System *54*
        Inflammation and Immune Function in Autism *55*
        Asthma *55*
    GI TRACT AND DIGESTION 55
        Digestive Function in Autism *55*
        Constipation *56*
        Hydrochloric Acid (HCl) *56*
    ENDOCRINE AND GLANDULAR FUNCTION 57
        Thyroid *57*
        Adrenals *58*
        Pancreas *59*
    TYING IT ALL BACK TO THE BRAIN 59
        Sleep *59*
        Seizures *60*
        Pyroluria *62*

PART TWO - COMPENDIUM OF NUTRITIONAL STRATEGIES AND OPPORTUNITY **63**

IMPACT OF NUTRIENTS **64**

    COMMON DEFICIENCIES 64
    DETERMINING DEFICIENCIES 65
        Assessments and Testing *66*
            GI Health Assessments 66
            Toxins and Detoxification Assessments 67
            Nutritional Status Assessments 68
            Hormones Assessments 68
            DNA Assessments 68
    GETTING STARTED WITH SUPPLEMENTS 69
    VITAMINS 70
        Vitamin A *70*
        Vitamin C *71*
        Vitamin E *72*
        Vitamin B6 .... *72*
        B6 and Magnesium *73*
        Vitamin B12 .... *73*
        Folic acid *74*
        Inositol *74*
        Biotin *74*
        Vitamin D *75*
        Vitamin K *76*
        Multivitamin/mineral formula *76*
    MINERALS 77
        Magnesium *77*
        Zinc *78*
        Calcium *79*
        Selenium *79*
    AMINO ACIDS 80
        DMG (Dimethylglycine) and TMG (Trimethylglycine) *80*
        NAC (N-acetyl cysteine) *80*
        Glutathione *81*
        Amino Acid Formulas *81*

ESSENTIAL FATTY ACIDS 83
    Omega-3 83
    Omega-6 and GLA 84
    Omega-9 84
    Fatty Acid Balance 84
GI SUPPLEMENTS 85
    Digestive Enzymes 85
    Probiotics... 87
    Butyric Acid 88
ADDITIONAL SUPPLEMENTS 88
    Colostrum 88
    Transfer Factors 88
    Phosphatidylcholine 89
    Medicinal Mushrooms 89
    Glyconutrients.. 89
    Coenzyme Q-10 (CoQ10) 90
    Pycnogenol 90
    Electrolytes 90
    Sulfates.. 90
    DMAE 91
    5-HTP (5-hydroxytryptophan) 91
    Adrenal Extract or Glandular 92
    Lectin Lock and NAG 92
    Melatonin... 92
    Herbs... 92
    Salt 94

ASD DIET OPTIONS **95**
    Gluten- and Casein-Free Diet (GFCF) 97
    Specific Carbohydrate Diet (SCD) 99
    The Body Ecology Diet 100
    Nourishing Traditions/Weston A. Price Diet (NT/WAP) 101
    Food Sensitivities... 102
    Elimination Diet... 103
    Rotation Diet.. 103
    Feingold Diet and Phenol Protocol... 104
    Low Oxalate Diet (LOD) 106
    Feast without Yeast 107
    Raw Food Diet... 108
    Paleolithic Diet.. 108
    Gut and Psychology Syndrome (GAPS) Diet.. 109
    Ketogenic Diet 109
    Coping with Picky Eaters 110

PART THREE - HOLISTIC GUIDE TO NUTRITION INTERVENTION............................. **112**

HOLISTIC NUTRITION APPROACH – STEP BY STEP **113**

#1 CLEANING UP THE DIET 116
    Artificial Ingredients/Food Additives 116
    MSG (Monosodium Glutamate)... 117
    Artificial Sweeteners 118
    Trans Fats and Hydrogenated Fats 119
    Pesticides 119
    Genetically Modified Organisms (GMOs).. 119
#2 CLEANING UP THE HOME 122
    Chlorine Bleach and other Chemical Cleaners 122

Perfumes or Fragrance...122
Building Materials and Solvents (paint, aerosols) 123
Fluoride..123
Fabric Softeners..123
Petroleum Jelly and Mineral Oil 124
Plastics/Phthalates..124
Cooking..124
#3 SUPPLEMENT BASICS...127
#4 DIET BASICS 128
Fat..129
Protein 132
    Grass-fed/Pastured Animal Foods 132
    Vegetarians and soy 133
Carbohydrates 133
    Sugar 133
#5 CHOOSING A FOUNDATIONAL ASD DIET 134
Gluten-free and Casein-Free 135
Specific Carbohydrate Diet: 136
Body Ecology Diet 136
Nourishing Traditions/Weston A. Price 137
Tips for the First Step of ASD Diet Implementation...137
#6 ADDRESSING FOOD INTOLERANCES: FOOD SENSITIVITIES AND PHENOLS...........138
Food Sensitivities/Allergies 138
    Assessing food sensitivities 139
    Food sensitivities and infants...140
Salicylates/Phenols 140
#7 EVOLVING THE DIET: NUTRITION BOOSTERS 141
Increasing the Quality of the Foods Your Child Already Eats....................................142
Sneaking Nutrients in the Diet, even with Picky Eaters. 143
    Nutrient-Dense Foods 143
    Mineral-rich Broths and Stocks 144
    Juicing...145
    Sneaking in Nutrients..146
Soaking and Fermenting..146
    Soaking and fermenting "seeds" 146
    Fermented foods..149
#8 REFINING THE ASD DIET 152
#9 CLEANING UP THE GUT...154
Balance Intestinal Flora and Support Digestion..154
Yeast (Candida) 155
Parasites..156
Supplements to Help the Gut 157
#10 SUPPLEMENT SPECIFICS...157
#11 SUPPORT IMMUNE FUNCTION 158
Viral/Bacterial Defense 158
Reducing Inflammation..159
#12 DETOXIFICATION 160
Supporting Detoxification...161
Chelation..162
Sweating and Far Infrared Sauna 164
PROGRESS AND REGRESSION...164

CONCLUSION...169

APPENDICES 170

    APPENDIX I - DEVELOPMENTAL CHARACTERISTICS OF AUTISM 171
    APPENDIX II - COMPARISON OF CHARACTERISTICS OF MERCURY POISONING & AUTISM 172
    APPENDIX III - POINTS TO CONSIDER FOR VACCINATION 175
    APPENDIX IV - YEAST DIET 177
    APPENDIX V - GLUTEN AND CASEIN FREE DIET 179
    APPENDIX VI – PARENTS RATINGS OF INTERVENTIONS 183
    APPENDIX VII - PHENOL PROTOCOL 184
    APPENDIX VIII - RAW DAIRY 187
    APPENDIX IX - SPECIFIC CARBOHYDRATE DIET (SCD) SUMMARY 192
    APPENDIX XI – SALICYLATES IN FOODS 194
    APPENDIX XIII - FAILSAFE DIET 198
    APPENDIX XIV - LOW OXALATE DIET (LOD) 200

RESOURCES 205

BIBLIOGRAPHY 210

INDEX 219

ABOUT THE AUTHOR 223

HOW TO READ THIS BOOK

I've intended for this book to be an informational resource, how-to guide, trusted reference, and workbook. In addition to gaining knowledge that will help you be the best advocate for your child, this book is a manual from which you can start helping right away while you determine questions you should ask your physician. Your nutrition approach for your child will evolve and change over time and as you return to this book, it will function as a great resource guide. I've included blank diet records, charts and lists you can copy and fill out or post on your refrigerator for reference.

This book will lay a foundation of knowledge, and then will take the reader on a tour of ideas that will be revisited again and again—often from different angles, or with fresh information. These concepts are complex and important, so I will be sharing them in small "bite-sized" pieces many times. You may also find it helpful to go back and reread sections. Each section is self-contained though builds from the previous section. Because of that, it's best to read this book from beginning to end the first time. After that, you can go back and skip around in any order.

If there is any information you find too complex, just read through it gaining as much information as you can. There have been many times in my studies that I read and listened to speakers four, five, or six times. It's amazing how much you will pick up by re-reading the information. When you return to it over time, you will have additional knowledge and a maturing perspective from which to see the information in a new light. If you prefer however, skip a section and come back to it later.

The book is referenced with parentheses and a bibliography versus endnotes. While I realize endnotes are more accepted in scientific texts, I prefer to view a list of all studies in order alphabetically by last name. This way I can look up a study by a particular researcher without having to know what page they are on. Thus, I have chosen to annotate the book this way.

Throughout the book I mention "children" with autism. This is because most parents begin their search for answers when their child is diagnosed; however, this book is for anyone on the autistic spectrum, including adults. Also, please note that while the sooner you intervene the quicker you'll see a response; this does not mean that older children and adults do not benefit. Anyone can benefit from nutritional intervention at any point in time.

I will be using the terms autism, autism spectrum disorders, and autistic spectrum disorder (ASD). Included within ASD are: autism, Asperger's Syndrome, low and high-functioning autism, PDD:NOS (Pervasive Developmental Disorder: Not Otherwise Specified), as well as ADHD (Attention Deficit Hyperactivity Disorder). Many do not want to think that ADHD is on the autism spectrum because of the stigma associated. I feel that only if we understand how these disorders are related and acknowledge the truth of the emerging information on this subject, can we do our best to help these children. As you read through this book, if you are interested in ADHD, please understand that what applies to ASD also applies to ADHD.

Diagnoses help us group disorders. Symptoms often overlap between diagnoses. Children with autism often have hyperactivity, inattentiveness—ADHD symptoms. Children with autism may also have aggression, irritability, anxiety, and other reactions. To me, the diagnosis is not as important as understanding how nutrition and diet affect these factors, and what can be done to relieve symptoms and aid healing. Many children with various diagnoses that involve behavior, mental/emotional health, learning disorders, sensory integration, tics and more can be helped by diet and the principles in this book.

With the rampant increase in childhood disorders around the globe, children with autism are the "canaries in the coalmine," alerting us and calling us to action. While the causes of the epidemic remain at issue, there is no doubt that helpful treatment approaches exist. Nourishing Hope involves applying the best nutrition principles and collective scientific knowledge to help our children heal. This information is applicable to varied health conditions facing children and adults today. These sound nutrition principles can help your whole family attain greater health and wellness for a lifetime.

PREFACE

S ince I began my professional studies in holistic nutrition and biochemistry, I have been particularly fascinated with nutrition for human development—that is, nutrition for children. From the onset, I investigated how artificial ingredients, low nutrient foods, and sugars were implicated in a wide range of newly epidemic disorders in children, particularly ADHD, type 2 diabetes ("adult-onset"), heart disease, and even autism.

Once I discovered that imbalanced biochemical pathways influence the symptoms of ADHD and autism and that food, nutrition, and proper supplementation can have significant impact on these disorders, I was drawn to learn and understand more. There are many people striving to help these children: parents, doctors, caregivers, educators, therapists, advocacy groups, nutritionists, researchers and research groups. If all of these people could better comprehend these factors and influences, we could use our collective knowledge to better help these children and their families. As I researched important subjects such as liver function, endocrine imbalance, the immune system, and food sensitivities, I would always ask the question, "How is this implicated in autism spectrum disorders, and how do we impact it through nutritional or supplemental interventions?"

Nourishing Hope is the culmination of seven years of research into and clinical experience with autism spectrum disorder and the affects of nutrition, environmental factors, and biochemical imbalances on these conditions. In this time, I have consulted with hundreds with children on the spectrum, read countless books and research papers, routinely attended (and now present at) leading conferences on the subject, interviewed leading-edge researchers, and collaborated with dozens of doctors and their patients.

My work continues steadfastly. I consult with parents and physicians through my office in San Francisco, and clients across the world by telephone. I am driven to share what I have learned and continue to learn. We all must share what we know so that all children on the spectrum and their families may harvest the life-bringing energies of hope. I believe that all people are worthy of (and deserve) hope—it is an inherently human capacity that, when nourished always leads to *some* positive outcome.

> **To Parents**: I hope this book will educate and empower your active role in choosing and co-creating with your health care practitioner the best path for your child. While we all need help and guidance, decisions regarding the direction to take with your child's health are uniquely personal. There is new, changing, and controversial information and only you can decide what directions you are willing to go. My desire is that this book will assist you in discussing information and strategizing approaches with your healthcare practitioners. It is for you, the courageous parents, and your children, that I press on in search of answers and more ways to help.

> **To Doctors**: I hope this book will inform you, your practice, and your efforts to help these children. You who are diligently on the front lines with these kids, their parents, and the many institutions trying both discover what is going on, and how to best provide help. I honor your work and intend to serve as best I can the continually emerging body

of knowledge and practice that nourishes hope for parents, practitioners, and the children we love.

To Nutrition and Holistic Colleagues: I hope this book inspires interest in applying your knowledge of health and healing in even broader ways. We are in this together. There are many children and families out there who need our help. May this book (and my experience and research) help further your work. Your experience, thoughts, and suggestions are welcome.

Please feel free to write to me: I am also open to your feedback on where to clarify, add, or correct information. Thank you for your support.

I wish you all the best on this path to healing. My desire is that this book will help you physically nourish yourselves and your children toward health, and nourish hope within you that there is a way, there is a path to healing.

Julie Matthews

INTRODUCTION

Autism has become an epidemic. In 2002, the UC Davis' M.I.N.D. Institute, in Sacramento, California found that the incidence of "full spectrum," or profound autism, had increased 273% in California from 1987 to 1998 and that this was "far in excess of population changes of approximately 20% for the State during the same time." (Bryd, 2002). Other states in America have also seen increases, as have many other countries. A 2001 study in Pediatrics reported a 1 in 250 incidence for full-spectrum autism in a New Jersey community (Bertrand: 2001) and a 2003 JAMA study found 1 in 294 in an Atlanta community, with a male to female ratio of 4:1 (Yeargin-Allsopp, 2003). In 2004, the CDC (Centers for Disease Control and Prevention) and the American Academy of Pediatrics published US statistics of 1 in 166 (CDC, 2004). Other countries, such as Sweden (Gillberg, 2006), Canada (Fombonne, 2006) and Australia (Icasiano, 2004) have also reported rises in the incidence of autism. In a 2006 *Lancet* report, Baird et al. state that 1 in 86 children in a community in England have ASD. (Baird, 2006). In most autism circles it is widely accepted that autism affects 1 in 150 children, and 1 in 94 boys.

Some critics continue to suggest that these findings are simply the result of better diagnostic techniques—since we can better identify ASD we find it more often. However, Dr. Robert S. Byrd, an epidemiologist and pediatrician at UC Davis states, "We wondered if the increase was real. Maybe we were doing a better job of finding causes. If the criteria for diagnosing autism had changed in those 10 years or if the definition had broadened, the mystery would be solved. But the standards used to diagnose full-spectrum autism were the same in both age groups." Further, he states, "You can't explain an increase of this magnitude on genetics. Something else is happening." (*NY Times*, 2002). Several DAN! Doctors, including David Traver M.D., have told me, "Genetics don't create epidemics."

Biochemical Imbalances Create a Neurological Disorder

Currently, the medical community defines autism as a psychiatric disorder, warranting a diagnosis using criteria found in *Diagnostic and Statistical Manual of Mental Disorders IV* (commonly called the *DSM-IV*). These criteria include impaired social interaction, impaired communication, and characteristic behavior patterns (See Appendix I). However, in spite of the fact that the diagnosis of autism stems from this manual, it is not a psychiatric, nor a psychological disorder. It is a *neurological* disorder. In other words, autism is a set of biochemical imbalances that create neurological/neurotransmitter imbalances, which result in psychological symptoms. In addition to the psychological (namely social and behavioral) symptoms; however, this faulty chemistry also manifests physical symptoms (See Appendix Ia).

The following are just some of the common biochemical imbalances among those with ASD that illustrate that autism is not just a "psychiatric disorder." According to William J. Walsh, Ph.D., founder and director of research of Health Research Institute and Pfeiffer Treatment Center, "more than 85% of untreated ASDs exhibit either severe zinc deficiencies or an elevated copper/zinc ratio," suggesting a metallathionein (MT) disorder and an inability to detoxify heavy metals. He suggests that the MT disorder also affects early brain development and the immune response and can result in GI problems. (Walsh, 2001). Jill James, Ph.D., found oxidative stress in children with autism including significantly lower baseline plasma concentrations of methionine, SAM, homocysteine, cystathionine, cysteine, and total glutathione than controls (James, 2004). This oxidative stress increases susceptibility to infection and inflammation—both seen in autism. You don't need to understand exactly what each of these conditions entails to see how they help to illustrate the biochemical imbalances behind this disorder and how these imbalances affect people psychologically (actually neurologically) and physically, creating the autistic traits we see.

There are no medical tests to determine autism, and the many physical symptoms are commonly ignored, even though it is known that those with autism share common physical symptoms. Acknowledging the physical symptoms is crucial—doing so shapes how we approach these disorders clinically and whether treatments are covered by medical insurance (parents spend tens of thousands of dollars out of pocket to address these biomedical issues that should be covered by insurance). Bryan Jepson, MD, of Thoughtful House, a treatment center for children with ASD, describes autism as "a disease of disordered biochemistry and metabolism that affects multiple organ systems, and it is treatable." (Jepson, 2007). The term biomedical is a popular term used to describe biochemical approaches to autism. While I do not practice medicine, as I am not a doctor, I do use some these biochemical (sometimes referred to as "biomedical") approaches and I have seen the positive outcomes and hope for the future they foster.

I've heard many stories of recovery including the wonderful story by Jenny McCarthy in her new book, *Louder Than Words: A Mother's Journey in Healing Autism*. In the words of late Bernard Rimland and the Autism Research Institute, "Recovery is possible."

PART ONE

Genetics, Environmental, and Biochemical Factors

The Etiology of Autism: Genetics and Environmental

In the vast majority of recent literature regarding autism, it is suggested that the etiology, or the cause, of autism is either genetic or environmental. That is, one has autism because genetic coding ordained it, or, conversely, because environmental assaults caused it. There is also a third, more comprehensive and plausible explanation: genetic weaknesses coupled with one or more environmental assaults results in the manifestation of autism (Deth). After years of personal research, conversations with hundreds of parents (including analysis of their presented test results and behavioral anecdotes), and dozens of interviews with practiced professionals in the field, it is this third explanation regarding the etiology of autism that I believe.

While there are genetic factors at play (later on I will discuss in more detail what research does tell us about genes and autism), I blame toxins as the major cause of autism. One of the reasons I believe toxins are a significant factor is the prevalence of regressive autism. According to Arthur Krigsman, MD, there are several "onsets" of autism: "early delay" is diagnosed very young at around six months and appears to be fairly rare; "regressive," where development progresses normally until around 18 to 24 months, at which time progress in language and social skills are lost; and "plateau" where development appears to have leveled out around age one, but over time it is evident that the child is actually slowly regressing (DAN! 2002). Many people, including myself, feel that regressive autism—the far more common type— illustrates the environmental etiology. This is because regressive autism is often very obvious— everything in the child is developing normally and then often out-of-the-blue things start to deteriorate and regress very quickly (sometimes overnight). In these cases, parents often share their stories of a single event such as an exposure to a vaccination causing high fever and loss of language, or a pesticide exposure causing seizures and the onset of autistic traits. In these cases we often see the "before and after" of an environmental assault having a significant impact. Lingam et al. in a 2003 study report that "27% of children with childhood autism had, by parental report, experienced regression" and "in 44 children with detailed records of regression, 42% had a specific trigger mentioned," with at least half of these triggers being a possible environmental assault. (Lingam, 2003). Geier et al. in 2007 found that eight of nine patients had regression and they feel that "evidence for mercury intoxication should be considered in the differential diagnosis as contributing to some regressive ASDs" (Geier, 2007). A 2007 report by the Vaccine Adverse Event Reporting System (VAERS), found that 19 out of 31 (61.3%) children "had evidence of developmental egression" (Woo, 2007).

According to the Autism Research Institute's website, "Prior to 1990, approximately two-thirds of autistic children were autistic from birth and one-third regressed sometime after age one year. Starting in the 1980's, the trend has reversed — fewer than one-third are now autistic from birth and two-thirds become autistic in their second year. The following results are based on the responses to ARI's E-2 checklist, which has been completed by thousands of autism families. These results suggest that something happened, such as increased exposure to an environmental insult, possibly vaccine damage, between ages 1 and 2 years."

While this increase in regressive autism points to an assault after birth, I don't want to leave out early onset as possibly being caused by environment as well. In these cases, because the event happens so early in life (perhaps during gestation) the effects of the exposure are not seen in the same way. Because in these cases the injury happens prior to or just after birth, it's not as easy to see the effect of the exposure as a "before and after." While this may lead people to believe that early onset is genetic (as the child seemed to be "born with it)," it may also be exposure of the mother to environmental factors such as the flu shot, rhogam, dental work which all affect the baby in utero, or the exposure to hepatitis B at birth.

While studying the differences between various "types" of autism may shed further light on the impact of genetics and environment, I feel that the information we have so far points to a genetic weakness (which is the reason every child doesn't end up with autism) coupled with one of these assaults at various points during development (creating regressive or early onset) that impacts children neurologically. The Autism Center at New Jersey Medical School-University of Medicine and Dentistry of New Jersey, Newark, supports the fact that genetic factors do seem to play a role in the cause of autism (Brimacombe, 2007).

Toxins Can Alter Genetics

Our world is highly toxic. There are tens of thousands of chemicals around us today that were not here even a few decades ago. These chemicals are not tested for safety with children or in combination with other chemicals (which we know makes them more toxic). In a study by the Environmental Working Group (EWG), researchers "found an average of 200 industrial chemicals and pollutants in umbilical cord blood from 10 babies born in August and September of 2004 in U.S. hospitals. Tests revealed a total of 287 chemicals in the group" (Environmental Working Group, 2005). The EWG study goes on to say that of the 287 chemicals, "180 cause cancer in humans or animals, 217 are toxic to the brain and nervous system, and 208 cause birth defects or abnormal development in animal tests."

In addition to chemicals being directly toxic to our bodies, these toxins can alter our genetics. Frank Gilliland, Professor of Preventative Medicine at the Keck School of Medicine in Los Angeles, and his colleagues conducted a study of epigenetics (or in this case transgenerational epigenetics)—the study of reversible, heritable changes in gene regulation that occur without a change in DNA sequence (genotype). The researchers believe that the toxins (in this case tobacco) may alter which genes are switched "on" or "off" in the fetus's reproductive cells, causing changes that are passed on to future generations. Gilliland found that children whose grandmothers smoked (not in front of the children) when pregnant had, on average, 2.1 times greater risk of developing asthma than children with grandmothers who never smoked. Even if the mother did not smoke, but the grandmother did, the child was still 1.8 times more likely to develop asthma. Whereas, if the mother smoked, the child was 1.5 times more likely to develop asthma than those born to non-smoking mothers. In other words, it was worse if grandmother smoked than if mother smoked.

It seems highly plausible that genetic susceptibility and epigenetics both play some role in the skyrocketing autism rates, but let us now examine more carefully the environmental assaults—which I believe are most implicated in autism—and how these assaults impact the biochemical pathways crucial to good health.

Environment and Biochemistry: Effects upon each other

Environmental assaults and biochemical pathways affect each other, often creating a vicious cycle. As you can see from the chart (Figure 1), environmental assaults can damage biochemistry and damaged biochemistry can inhibit our ability to handle environmental assaults. The chart illustrates the complexity of the causes and contributing factors involved in ASD (each component of the chart will be explained later in the book). As you can see, many factors contribute to the malfunction of other areas, creating a downward spiral of events. In another example, yeast overgrowth, inflammation, and a very restricted diet can lead to a further weakened immune system. The cycles are vicious.

Some of the major systems affected in ASD are digestion, detoxification, and immune function. Poor digestion contributes to nutrient deficiencies, the creation of food sensitivities leading to further inflammation and digestion problems, the creation of toxins from dysbiotic bacteria that affect the brain, the production of opiates from food that affect brain function. Poor detoxification overloads the system leading to further toxicity—toxins cause direct damage and inflammation to the brain, damage digestion, damage biochemical pathways, and can influence genetic expression. Poor immune function can cause reliance on antibiotics damaging the gut, gut flora, and digestion, weakens the ability to fight viruses and yeast, and creates inflammation.

Inflammation appears to be involved in most of these systems. Toxins increase inflammation. Dysregulated immune function causes inflammation to go awry. Gut permeability and increased food reactions creates gut and systemic inflammation. Yeast overgrowth, a result of poor immune function, creates inflammation and contributes to further digestive insufficiency. Faulty sulfation and reduced glutathione production, both important components of our detoxification system, increase inflammation.

In fact, inflammation may be at the center of autism. Inflammation in other parts of the body can create inflammation in the brain. Richard Lathe, the author of over 100 peer-reviewed journal articles, describes in detail in his book *Autism, Brain, and Environment* how inflammation in the body affects inflammation in the brain. Lathe states, "GI tract inflammation can signal directly to the limbic brain, stimulating local toxic cytokine (regulates inflammation) production and neuronal damage" (Lathe, 2006). As Lathe points out, infections including respiratory infection (from pertussis), dysentery causing bacteria (shigella dysenteriae), and pertussis vaccine have been shown to elevate inflammatory markers in the brain. (Loshcher, 2000; Nofech-Mozes, 2000; and Donnelly 2001). A study by Vargus, et al. in the *Annals of Neurology* discovered a "unique proinflammatory profile of cytokines" in the brain indicating "innate neuroimmune reactions play a pathogenic role in an undefined proportion of autistic patients" (Vargas, 2005).

While science does not yet fully understand the exact interplay between genetic, biochemical and environmental factors, what is clear is that they are all involved and the picture is complex. They seem to fuel each other, often creating further problems for an already burdened system.

11

Figure 1: Underlying Causes and Contributors to ASD

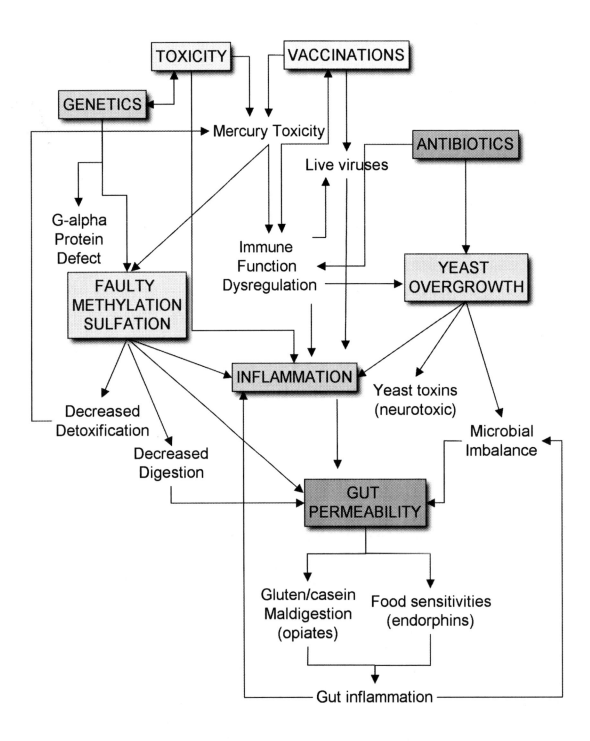

GENETICS

No one has pinpointed one genetic cause of autism, and I don't feel we will find ONE genetic cause. Studies on twins support this notion. If the disorder were purely genetic, monozygotic twins would both be autistic, 100% of the time. In actuality however, there is only a 60% concordance rate between monozygotic twins and an 86% concordance rate of the second twin having some features of autism or associated disorders (Risch et al, 1999).

Several teams of researchers speculate which chromosomal sites may be affected in autism although these speculations differ greatly and nothing has been proven or is consistent to date. The chromosomes researched and suspected include chromosomes 1 and 17 (Risch et al, 1999), 7q and 16p (IMGSAC, 1998), 2q and 17q (IMGSAC, 2001), 6q and 7q (Phillipe et al, 1999), 13q and 7q.

A small number of individuals with ASD have a specific genetic metabolic fault that has autism as one of its manifestations. Some include Fragile X, Phenylketonuria (PKU) or hyperhhenylalaninuria, histidinemia/histidinuria, Lesch-Nyhan syndrome. I will not be focusing on these causes of autism. However, even with these genetic factors, there is more going on than just genetics, as the "prevalence rates of autism in Fragile X have been estimated at 15–33%" (Kaufmann, 2004)

Polymorphisms (differences in DNA sequences among individuals) involving several methylation processes (pathways known to be impaired in autism) have been identified in higher numbers with people with autism. Identifying these polymorphisms may prove helpful as they are being used as indicators of autism risk.

We often think of genetics as fixed, that is, you have a particular gene and you're stuck with what manifests. There is no changing it. However, there is much more to genetics. Genetic factors do not always affect the DNA sequence itself (as we often think). Epigenetics is the study of heritable changes in gene function that occur without a change in the sequence of the DNA. DNA methylation, is the best-understood epigenetic markers to date that affects this expression of the gene, without changing the DNA sequencing itself. (You'll notice that term methylation again, it's even so important that it affects gene expression.)

Gene expression can be influenced by toxic exposure and nutrients (or nutrient deficiencies). Nutrogenomics is the study of the effect of nutrients on health through altering genome (genes) and the resulting changes in physiology. In other words, both toxic exposure and healthful nutrients can significantly impact our epigenetics, or who we become to some degree.

Duke University researchers, Jirtle and Waterland, in their agouti mice study showed that diet can dramatically alter heritable phenotypic change in agouti mice, not by changing DNA sequence but by changing the DNA methylation pattern of the mouse genome. (Waterland, 2003) This study (discussed in detail below) is a wonderful example of the power and interplay between diet and genetic expression within a single generation of offspring—as Jirtle says, "where environment interfaces with genomics."

Parents and practitioners should know that there are things one can do to positively affect autism, even if "it is genetic."

In terms of toxins interfering with genetics, we see Mary Megson's work on how a pertussis toxic appears to alter the g-alpha protein. (Megson, 2000). A 2007 study in the *Journal of Neurological Sciences* found that "transient intrauterine deficits of thyroid hormones (as brief as three days) result in permanent alterations of cerebral cortical architecture reminiscent of those observed in brains of patients with autism" and suggest that the "current surge of autism could be related to transient maternal hypothyroxinemia resulting from dietary and/or environmental exposure to antithyroid agents" such as goitrogens, herbicides, polychlorinated biphenyls (PCBs), perchlorates, mercury, and coal derivatives such as resorcinol, phthalates, and anthracenes. (Roman, 2007).

G-Alpha Protein Defect

A G-alpha protein defect is a genetic defect characterized by night blindness and various parathyroid, thyroid, and pituitary gland conditions. Mary Megson found those with a family history of at least one parent with a G-alpha protein defect are more likely to have a child who develops autism (Megson, 2000). The data suggest that a toxin separates the G-alpha protein from the retinoid receptors in the hippocampus by depleting the store of vitamin A.

Megson's work supports the theory that autism is (frequently) a combination of genetic background combined with environmental assault. A G-alpha protein defect, which runs in families, combined with the environmental assault of pertussis toxin from the DTP vaccination, appears to be causing autism.

On a positive note on how we can affect our genetic expressions through diet, Megson noticed that supplementation with vitamin A from cod liver oil has a positive impact on these children, particularly in regard to language and vision. She believes the vitamin A may reconnect the retinoid receptors, which are essential for vision, sensory perception, language processing, and attention.

Polymorphisms Associated with Methylation

We are beginning to understand the polymorphisms (differences in DNA sequences) that play some role in autism. Several that we know about currently include: MTHFR, RFC, TCN2, CBS, and GST. Interestingly, each of these polymorphisms has an effect on methylation or transsulfuration, the biochemical pathways that when functioning improperly play a crucial role in autism.

These enzymes have important functions in the body, and if polymorphisms are expressed in a way to diminish these healthy functions, you can see the possible biochemical processes that can go awry—many of which we do see in autism. MTHFR (5,10-methylenetetrahydrofolate reductase) is an enzyme in folate metabolism that facilitates the formation of methyltetrahydrofolate (methyl-THF), a required cofactor in the remethylation of homocysteine to methionine. CBS (cystathionine beta synthase) is an enzyme, which regulates the conversion of homocysteine to cystathionine (and down the transsulfuration) pathway). GST (glutathione S-transferase) is responsible for detoxifying certain products of oxidative stress and a variety of electrophilic xenobiotics and carcinogens (Genovations.com). GSTM1 is primarily located in the liver, where as GSTP1 is located primarily in the brain and lungs. Each of these enzymes has been identified as having a polymorphism.

Interestingly, the above polymorphisms involve methylation, and poor methylation can affect DNA through gene expression. Poor methylation affects many of the biochemical pathways that are impaired with autism and they are important processes to understand so parents and physicians can guide nutritional and supplement intervention. We will be studying these in detail in the next section.

Other Polymorphisms

In addition to polymorphisms that affect methylation, there are other polymorphisms that affect detoxification and important biochemistry in autism in other ways – SOD, COMT, and GABRB3 are three of these. SOD (superoxide dismutase) is an antioxidant enzyme that converts reactive oxygen species into hydrogen peroxide. It's a suspected contributor in ASD and Down syndrome.

COMT (catechol-O-Methyltransferase) is a key enzyme involved in the deactivation of catechol compounds, estrogens, various chemicals and toxins. In the brain, COMT modulates neurotransmitter functions. GABRB3, is a polymorphism in the GABA receptor (that according to wikipedia is associated with savant skills). The GABRB3 is a "type A receptor b3 subunit has been associated with autism in two studies" (Veenstra-VanDerWeele, 2003).

Epigenetics and DNA Methylation

Epigenetics is the process of changing the gene expression without changing the DNA. DNA methylation is the most understood and studied area of epigenetics. When a methylated DNA sequence replicates, only one strand of the next-generation double helix has all its methyl markers intact; the other strand needs to be remethylated. DNA methylation is a way of propagating the genomic pattern from one generation to the next. Because a genome can pick up or drop a methyl group more easily than changing the DNA sequence, it is a quick way for an organism, as Jirtle says, "to respond to the environment without having to change its hardware."

The agouti mice have been the source of several studies of epigenetics, DNA methylation, and the effects of methyl supplementation. Agouti is a dominant gene that gives mice yellow fur (just as brown eyes are a dominant gene in humans but someone can have blue, green or brown – yellow is the dominant gene for the mice fur)—and the mice are either yellow, brown, or some mix of the two. When Waterland and Jirtle fed folic acid, vitamin B12, choline, and betaine (methyl donor supplements) to the pregnant mice, their offspring had mostly brown fur (instead of the dominant yellow), and more importantly were not highly susceptible to obesity, diabetes, and cancer (Waterland and Jirtle, 2003). Mice without the methyl-rich nutrients had mostly yellow pups and a much higher susceptibility to obesity, diabetes, and cancer. These changes resulted even though all the offspring inherited exactly the same agouti gene. Waterland and Jirtle (Waterland and Jirtle, 2004) provide evidence that DNA methylation might be the critical link by which nutritional deficiencies during early pregnancy might cause chronic diseases in the adult.

Although it seems a bit backwards, methylation turns *off* genes (taking off methyl groups turns them on); however, in some cases, as this one, we want to turn off some genes for our health. Additionally, methylation turned off gene expression in the test mice as well as their offspring. In another study in 2006, Waterland states "Methyl donor supplementation of female mice before and during pregnancy permanently increases DNA methylation…in the offspring" (Waterland, Dolinoy, et al, 2006). In this study, Waterland and his team observed a tail-specific change that suggests hypermethylation occurred mid-term, showing that dietary influence is "not limited to early embryonic development." In a second study in 2006 Waterman used methionine to affect DNA methylation and states, "Nutrition during diverse stages of life can influence epigenetic gene regulation (Waterland, 2006).

There is a lot of great clinical work being done by doctors like Lawrence G. Leichtman, M.D. who are helping parents work on methylation for gene expression in future children.

DNA methylation might be the critical link by which nutritional deficiencies during early pregnancy might change gene expression and causing changes in biochemistry pathways and lead to diseases such as autism. While much more research needs to be done on epigenetics, this study shows the beginning of understanding how nutrition and deficiencies influence genetic expression. It also begs the question as to whether other environmental factors such as toxins might also influence genetic expression that can be passed to offspring.

While there are practitioners who use genetic testing to guide intervention, results with this approach are mixed. I'm pointing out these polymorphisms and their related effects on biochemistry to show how genetics are involved and how complicated this can be. As we begin to know more and more, this information will become more useful in guiding intervention.

Family History and Common Disorders

The field of genetics is in its early stages and there is much we do not know yet. As such, I wanted to include a discussion on connections that have been made between disorders that run in families—hinting at a link to genetics. While we may not have found the "gene that causes autism" (I don't think we will ever find only *one*), what we have learned so far with genetics and how it effects biochemistry helps support the connection between common disorders we see running in families with autism.

The following are neurological and autoimmune conditions that appear to run in families with autism.

Disorders Running in Families

Neurological Disorders	**Autoimmune/Inflammatory Diseases**
Autism	Lupus
ADHD	Rheumatoid arthritis
Tourette's	Hoshimoto's/hypothyroid
Asperger's	Type 1 diabetes
Depression	Chronic fatigue
Schizophrenia	Fibromyalgia
Bipolar	Crohn's disease

Neurological disorders appear to run in families. It's common in my practice to see children with autism have a parent with ADHD or another family member with schizophrenia or Tourette's. In a study of Tourette's and ADHD, researchers found a significant association with tics and ADHD, finding "of the relatives with Tourette's Syndrome, 61% had ADD and 36% had ADHD. Of the relatives with chronic tics, 41% had ADD and 26% had ADHD" (Knell, 1993).

One of the commonalities between the neurological and inflammatory groups above is with the biochemistry of sulfation (or faulty sulfation). Dr. Ben Feingold, Chief Immunologist and Allergist at Kaiser Permanente in San Francisco in the 1970's, was one of the first to recognize great similarities between ADHD and autism. Dr. Feingold noticed that certain artificial ingredients (phenols, to be discussed later) made some children inattentive, hyperactive, and display autistic-like symptoms. This inability of those with autism to process phenols, which we now have seen through research such as that done by Rosemary Waring, is most likely due to faulty sulfation. Sinzig, et al report many common symptoms between autism and ADHD, such as "hyperactivity, impulsivity and attention deficit disorder." (Sinzig et al, 2007). Additionally, Dr. David Comings, of City of Hope Medical Center in Duarte, CA has found the coexistence in families of ADHD with Tourette's syndrome (Comings, 2001, Knell, et al, 1993)

Faulty sulfation may be one link between ASDs and autoimmune as Rosemary Waring's (Ph.D., Biosciences, University of Birmingham, UK) work shows. She discovered that 71% of those with lupus had impaired sulfoxidation and 60% had no sulfoxides compared with 36% and 4% respectively in a control population; (Waring, 1992:25). Those with rheumatoid arthritis have less capacity to excrete the non-toxic conjugate of paracetamol (acetominophen), pointing to poor sulfate detoxification (Waring, 1991:689). As Waring also found that children with autism have faulty sulfation, it seems logical that the same genetic tendency (possibly something similar to the polymorphisms associated with methylation) is expressed differently with different people—and is likely dependent on environmental factors. These studies by Waring show that the autoimmune conditions (lupus and rheumatoid arthritis) and autism involve faulty sulfation (described later), and support Comi's findings of autoimmune disorders and autism running in families. When we discuss the environmental triggers and biochemistry of methylation and sulfation later, you will see some of the reasons why this connection is not only plausible, but likely.

Autoimmune disorders and autism have been well researched by other researchers as well. Dr. Ann M. Comi of John Hopkins Hospital, Department of Neurology, found a link between autoimmune disorders and autism. Out of 61 autistic parents, 46% had two or more family members with autoimmune disorders, most common being type 1 diabetes, adult rheumatoid arthritis, hypothyroidism, and systemic lupus erythematosus (Comi, 1999:388). When there were three or more family members with an autoimmune disorder, the likelihood of autism increased 5.5 times, and when the mother of a subject had an autoimmune disorder, likelihood increased 8.8 times (Comi, 1999:388). A 2007 study found that two autoimmune conditions were associated with autism: ulcerative colitis in mothers and type 1 diabetes in fathers. (Mouridsen et al, 2007).

You can begin to see how similar underlying physiology could cause any of the neurological diseases seen on this spectrum. Most likely the appearance of different neurological diseases depends on the unique environmental factors and the age at which these factors occur.

Research shows a link between ADHD and depression in the mothers of children with autism. L.E. McCormick, M.D. found in 1995 that there is a link between mothers with depression and a child with ADHD (McCormick, 1995). Another study in 1997 by Stephen Foraone, Ph.D., and Joseph Beiderman, M.D. uncovered overwhelming evidence of a familial link between ADHD and depression (Foraone and Beiderman, 1997:533). It seems fair to extrapolate from this a possible connection between mothers with depression and children with autism. This intrigues me, as many of the families I work with have a history of depression, especially mothers. While I have not done a formal survey, in my practice, a significant number of mothers with children on the spectrum have told me about their depression. There was a period of time where around 70% of mothers I worked with had pretty significant depression, including some on antidepressants. It was frustrating that many doctors dismissed these mothers with comments such as, "Of course you are depressed, your child has autism" when these mothers had experienced depression since their college days, long before having kids.

In spite of genetic frailties, children on the autism spectrum can recover, as can others in the family who struggle with neurological and autoimmune conditions. By addressing nutritional and biochemical support, environmental factors, and using other holistic interventions, improved health is very possible.

ENVIRONMENTAL FACTORS and BIOCHEMICAL IMPACT

Mercury Toxicity

Mercury is a highly toxic substance. It is known to create brain damage in children and can cause death even if exposure is relatively small. We are exposed to mercury in different ways and in different forms, and some are more dangerous than others.

Types of Mercury

Three different types of mercury exist, varying in their levels of toxicity. They are elemental mercury, inorganic mercury and organic mercury. The California Poison Control System (http://www.calpoison.org/public/mercury.html) and ATSDR (Agency for Toxic Substances and Disease Registry) (http://www.atsdr.cdc.gov/mercury/) provide the following information on the various forms and sources of mercury:

1) Elemental mercury (Hg0)
   - Also known as metallic mercury or liquid mercury and is an extremely heavy, odorless, silver colored liquid
   - Exists as a natural element in the earth's crust and is released into the air by natural processes, such as volcanic activity.
   - Common sources in the home include broken mercury thermometers, broken fluorescent light bulbs, dental amalgam fillings and mercury containing latex paints
   - Metallic mercury is also released into the environment (primarily into air) from mining, smelting, industrial activities, combustion of fossil fuels (such as coal)
   - Toxicity is mainly caused by inhalation of elemental mercury vapors, as mercury is well absorbed by the lungs. To develop problems by inhalation you need either a large one-time exposure or a long-term exposure. Elemental mercury not absorbed from the stomach and will not cause any poisoning in a healthy person, nor is it well absorbed across the skin.

2) Inorganic mercury
   - Are known as mercuric salts and mercuric chloride, mercuric iodide etc
   - Sources are calomel and cinnabar, certain Chinese herbal ball preparations and some Indian and Mexican folk medications
   - Organic mercury is also released into the environment (primarily into air) from mining, smelting, industrial activities, combustion of fossil fuels (such as coal)
   - Is extremely toxic when ingested and damages the kidneys

3) Organic mercury
   - Organic mercury passes into the breast milk
   - Ethylmercury
     - Are found in a variety of products and are used medically as fungicides and antibacterials
     - Common sources in the home are mercurochrome (merbromin) and merthiolate (thimerosal)
   - Methylmercury
     - Another source of organic mercury is the ingestion of mercury-contaminated food, usually fish. Microorganisms in the environment can convert inorganic mercury (from the environment) to the organic form methylmercury. When lake, river or ocean water is contaminated with methylmercury compounds, the mercury accumulates and magnifies

in the flesh of the fish. Organic mercury concentrations can be more than 1,000 times greater in the fish than in the surrounding water

- Oral and intestinal bacteria can methylate mercury to methyl-mercury (Haley: 2002)

Effects of Mercury

Mercury is a highly toxic substance. Mercury enters the body and what is not excreted can travel to the brain, change to inorganic mercury, cling to brain tissue and damage the nervous system. Once mercury has changed to inorganic mercury, it is virtually impossible for the body to excrete it naturally, that is, without some sort of help. Mercury lodges in the exact part of the brain damaged in autism, so the effects on the brain (symptoms) are almost identical between mercury toxicity and autism.

Additionally, we know from past experience of pink disease (where the mercury in teething powder sickened (and in some cases killed) hundreds of babies and Minimata Disease (where water contaminated with mercury in Japan sickened and killed hundreds of people) that only about one in 500 are often severely affected by mercury. Boyd Haley, Ph.D., Professor and Chair of the Department of Chemistry, University of Kentucky, says that reaction to mercury varies greatly in the population (DAN! 2002). Bernard states that mercury poisoning among individuals varies greatly depending on dose, type of mercury, method of exposure, duration, and individual sensitivity (Bernard, 2001:462)—explaining why some individuals may develop autism from vaccine mercury exposure, and others do not.

Dr. Haley has done extensive research on mercury toxicity as it relates to Alzheimer's disease and ASD. Haley has observed that mercury in thimerosal (the sort common in vaccinations up until a few years ago, and still used in some) is more toxic than mercury from environmental exposure (Hg2+) and both forms significantly reduce tubulin, part of the neuron that causes the cessation of neurite process growth (DAN! Syllabus, 2002:246). Additionally, the toxicity of thimerosal is increased in the presence of aluminum (found in many vaccines), as well as testosterone (DAN! Syllabus, 2002:246). In fact, during a particular experiment of Dr. Haley's, 5% neuron death was observed with exposure to thimerosal in culture, whereas 100% cell death occurred with the addition of a non-toxic concentration of testosterone (DAN! Syllabus, 2002:246). Additionally, estrogen was found to be protective against mercury toxicity. This may account for the 4:1 difference we see between boys and girls who develop autism (Lotspeich, 1993:87).

Mercury in Autism

Bernard, et al., points to this causal relationship between mercury poisoning and autism based on a stong similarity between characteristics of mercury poisoning and autism, as well as biological abnormalities that occur in both (Bernard, 2001:462), see Appendix II. Those diagnosed with mercury poisoning and autism share these characteristics (among others):
- Arm flapping, rocking, and walking on toes
- Oversensitive to sound and touch
- Failure to develop speech
- Poor eye contact
- Decreased muscle tone and sleeping difficulties

The degree of similarity is so striking between mercury poisoning and autism that a causal relationship cannot be ignored. Then the question arises, "Is autism as simple as mercury poisoning?" In some cases I suppose mercury poisoning could be misdiagnosed as autism. However, most often, I'd say it's more complex. There are many factors involved with autism of which mercury can play a big role. Mercury exposure has such wide-ranging and disruptive powers that it certainly can be powerful enough to kickstart a downward cascade of biochemical and physiological problems that can lead someone into autism. Mercury cannot be ignored as a cause in autism but it is also not the only factor.

Boyd Haley, Ph.D., in his testimony before the House Government Reform Committee in 2002, stated that individuals with autism are "much more susceptible to neurological damage through exposures to mercury" because they "are not effective at excreting mercury." (Haley, 2002). A 2007 study by Geier et al, looked at the relationship between ASD and prenatal mercury exposure from thimerosal-containing Rho(D)-immune globulins and found that "prenatal mercury exposure may play" a role "in some children with ASDs" (Geier:2007).

Those with ASD often show significantly higher levels of mercury and other heavy metals in their systems. Bradstreet et al. studied the level of mercury excreted with a three-day oral challenge with the heavy metal chelator DMSA (Bradstreet 2003). Bradstreet found that the children with autism had significantly higher levels of urinary excretion of mercury upon chelation. The control group and the unvaccinated groups showed equally low levels of mercury, suggesting that neurotypical children were able to excrete the mercury from the vaccination, unlike the children with ASD.

Additionally, mercury is known to cling to the brain and tissues (and not be excreted in the urine or present in the hair) so tests can fail to indicate high mercury levels even when it is present. Holmes' research highlights this well. Holmes et al. studied children with autism against control children without autism, all who had been fully vaccinated, and found that there was a significant difference in the levels of mercury (Holmes 2003). Initially, the results were confusing as they found lower levels of mercury in the hair tests of those with autism, when they expected to find higher levels. They noticed that the lowest levels were present in those with the highest exposure to mercury; moreover, these children were also the most severely autistic. However, upon further reflection, it became clear that hair is a measure of what the body is able to naturally *detoxify,* as hair is one excretory system our body employs. While the study was not methodologically flawless, it strongly suggests that poor detoxification could be a factor in autism and traditional testing methods may not catch toxicity, hence clinicians and researchers may be unaware of toxins and mercury as a cause for autism and are not giving it the attention and research it deserves.

If most children are immunized, then why don't most children have high levels of mercury or mercury poisoning? One answer lies in the individual's ability to detoxify the mercury—one possibility is faulty sulfation and poor methylation. Additional reasons for individual variance include time of development for exposure, sex of child and hormones present, antibiotic use, other toxic exposures, overburden of the liver, and the combination of factors happening simultaneously. Any or all of these factors can impact the body's ability to detoxify mercury causing some individuals to store this mercury and become mercury poisoned. As we will see, mercury not only causes severe damage to the brain and other body systems, but also to the biochemical process that would normally aid the detoxification of mercury. This causes a "double whammy" (seen so often in ASD), allowing for the build up of these toxins while disabling the systems that could help eliminate it.

In addition to causing brain damage, mercury can damage the immune system. With autism, we often see decreased immune function. Thimerosal (ethylmercurithiosalicylate) inhibits DPP-IV (dipeptidylpeptidase IV) an enzyme needed to break down gluten and casein. In addition to breaking down gluten and casein, DPP-IV influences T cells (cell-mediated immune system cells that are directed primarily at microbes) in the immune system and is a binding protein for purine and adenosyl deaminase (enzyme involved in purine metabolism with an important role in energy regulation). As such, low DPP-IV can impair the immune system, unbalance amino acids, and attenuate methylation. Thimerosal can also impair immune response by damaging lymphocytes via deoxyadenosine, and can impair physiologic methylation (Pangborn and Baker, 2001:54). In a nutshell, mercury inhibits DPP-IV, CD26 and ADABP. The effects of inhibition of these substances match the symptoms of autism (Pangborn and Baker, 2001:55).

While mercury is highly toxic and damaging to the brain and biochemistry, it is possible to detoxify mercury. Upon detoxification, children experience a reduction in symptoms, begin to heal, and can even recover from autism.

Sources of Exposure

Exposure to heavy metals may be from direct contact or through the mother. A child can be exposed to heavy metals from vaccinations, chewing on lead-based painted toys, and other environmental sources. Children may also be exposed through their mother's exposure during pregnancy with the child or while nursing, or from a mother's body burden before getting pregnant that exposes the fetus to the toxins in her system.

Amalgams

Amalgam fillings (which are 50% mercury) are a common source of mercury, most especially if placed in or removed from the mother prior to conception, during pregnancy, or while nursing. Amalgam fillings in the child would also be a mercury source. Not only does the individual get large exposures upon placing the amalgam fillings but also the continued off gassing of mercury vapor that is inhaled with chewing and breathing. Boyd Haley, a well-known researcher on mercury toxicity and the negative affects on the brain in Alzheimer's and autism states, "Mercury vapors, released in the mouth from dental amalgams, have been proven to be the most readily absorbed form of mercury by the human body. 80% of inhaled mercury vapors are retained by the body" (mercurypoisoned.com).

A Swedish study analyzed the "results of removing dental amalgam in 15 studies each with more than 20 patients, published during the years 1986-1997." Clinical improvements were seen in 37 to 97% of patients and "antibody titers in patients with autoimmune diseases diminished" (Berglund).

While other countries such as Canada and Sweden are banning or strongly recommending against amalgams being placed in pregnant and nursing mothers or children, the United States is denying any problem with amalgams. Health Canada, the Federal department responsible for helping Canadians maintain and improve their health suggests on their website (www.hc-sc.gc.ca), "when the fillings need to be repaired, you may want to consider using a product that does not contain mercury. Pregnant women, people allergic to mercury and those with impaired kidney function should avoid mercury fillings. Children should be filled with non-mercury materials" (Health Canada, 1996). Tragically, the United States is not making these recommendations.

Diet

Our diet is another source of exposure of mercury (methylmercury) from fish and other seafood. On the EPA's website they state, "For fetuses, infants, and children, the primary health effect of methylmercury is impaired neurological development." While some fish such as salmon appear to be in a safe range for *adults*, others such as swordfish have a level of 150 mcg, or more—and for children, pregnant women, and children with autism, there may not be a safe limit based on their size and/or detoxification function. Fish with the highest levels of methylmercury are mackerel king, shark, swordfish and tilefish, with levels of 0.7 PPM (parts per million) to 4.5 PPM. Bass, marlin, halibut, tuna and orange roughy also have relatively high levels, with 0.1 PPM to 2.1 PPM. Because of the complication to convert parts per million to micrograms, there are calculators available to determine a safe limit based on body weight and type of fish. One such resource is www.GotMercury.org. The website http://www.cfsan.fda.gov/~frf/sea-mehg.html has the complete list of all fish and their levels (U.S. Department of Health and Human Services and U.S. Environmental Protection Agency, 2006). However, this calculation does not take age, size of individual, detoxification capability, or pregnancy into consideration.

The FDA currently has advice for consumers (posted on the Internet) recommending that pregnant women, and women of childbearing age who may become pregnant, limit their consumption of shark and swordfish to no more that one meal per month (FDA 1998) because of the extreme levels. Consumption of high mercury fish during pregnancy causes an immediate exposure and threat to the fetus. Additionally, for a woman of childbearing age that can not detoxify and excrete mercury as effectively as the general population consumption of fish high in mercury can result in accumulation of mercury in her system before she gets pregnant, creating exposure of mercury to the fetus. Xue et al reported in Environmental Health Perspective that fish consumption was "positively associated with higher mercury levels in hair" and increased the risk of preterm delivery (before 35 weeks). "The greatest fish source for mercury exposure appeared to be canned fish," with 25% of the women eating greater than 12 fish meals in a 6 month period (Xue, 2007). Unfortunately the study does not mention what type of canned fish was consumed. Hsu et al, looking at fish consumption in Taiwanese pregnant women, report that "total mercury concentrations of maternal blood, cord blood and placenta tissue commonly exceeded recommended values, and were higher in women who ate fish more than three times a week while pregnant" (Hsu, 2007).

Although certain types of fish contain high amounts of methylmercury, there is some discrepancy – in may not be necessary for all people to exclude all fish their diet. Some perspective is necessary. A 2003 Swedish study found no association between fish consumption and methylmercury in cord blood but did determine that inorganic mercury in cord blood "increased significantly with increasing number of maternal dental amalgam fillings." (Björnberg, 2003) Boyd Haley, Ph. D, in his testimony before the House Government Reform Committee in 2002, states that the "fact that amalgams are most likely the major contributor to the mercury levels in American citizens should be clearly presented to the public. Yet all the American public hears is concerns about mercury in fish" (Haley, 2002). In an interview on Autism One Radio in 2006, Boyd Haley Ph.D reaffirms that "exposing yourself to mercury that's already bound up with selenium, bound up with other protective compounds that you find in the fish—is totally different than mercury coming off of a dental amalgam. The one is excreted rapidly and the other one is not." Haley believes that "over 90% of the mercury in the bodies of mothers who give birth to autistic children, and in the blood of not only the mother but anybody else that has amalgam fillings" comes from (mercury off gassing) their dental amalgams (with an average of four or five amalgam fillings) (Haley, 2006).

It appears we can deal with mercury much better from food than from other sources of exposure. While the mercury in fish is certainly problematic for some, it appears to be a convenient scapegoat for all of our mercury toxicity. However, children with high heavy metal loads or are poor detoxifiers should still avoid fish.

Air

Air pollution is another important source of mercury (and other toxins). There are two significant studies illustrating poorer air quality is related to increased rates of autism. The first was a study done by Palmer et al. in which they investigated the relationship between mercury in the air and rates of autism from data from Texas Education Department and the United States Environmental Protection Agency. They found "for each 1,000 lb of environmentally released mercury, there was a 43% increase in the rate of special education services and a 61% increase in the rate of autism. (Palmer, 2006). The second study was done in the San Francisco Bay Area by Windham et al. They found a 50 % increase in autism in areas with the top quartile or highest levels of chlorinated solvents and heavy metals, mainly mercury, cadmium, nickel, trichloroethylene, and vinyl chloride (Windham, 2006). Windham concluded, "Our results suggest a potential association between autism and estimated metal concentrations, and possibly solvents, in ambient air around the birth residence."

Vaccines and what they used to contain

Since the 1930's, most vaccinations contained thimerosal, an inexpensive preservative containing 49.6% ethylmercury (Bernard, 2001:462). While very recently the mercury has finally been removed for the most part from childhood vaccines in America and Europe, millions of children were affected during the decades when large amounts of mercury were used in vaccines. Thimerosal is still used in vaccines in many countries and a Brazilian study published in September 2007 speculates that the amount of thimerosal ethylmercury exposure from the vaccines "modulated the relative increase in hair-mercury of breast-fed infants at six months of age" (Marques, 2007).

Thimerosal in vaccines was and is injected directly into the blood stream bypassing many of the body's natural defense systems, like the gut. Mercury can then cross the blood brain barrier and lodge in brain tissue, causing brain damage. Additionally, babies are essentially defenseless to detoxify it. Bile, which helps clear toxins from the body, is not produced in infants until after 4-6 months of life (Cave, 2001: 62). According to the EPA, the "safe" level of mercury, assuming a proper functioning detoxification system is .1 mcg per kilogram of body weight per day (Cave, 2001:62). Until the removal of thimerosal from the vaccines, just one hepatitis vaccine had 12.5 micrograms of mercury; this is <u>25 times</u> the EPA's safe level (Cave, 2001, 62). With these older mercury-containing vaccines, by the age six of months an infant had received 187.5 micrograms of mercury from their childhood vaccinations! How could all of these vaccinations, in such a short period of time, *not* increase an infant's mercury level to extremely toxic amounts!

Additionally, vaccinations are given to pregnant women and nursing women. Until recently, Rhogam (for Rh-negative women) contained mercury and the fetus was exposed to the mercury through this vaccine. Today the flu shot still contains mercury. Given while the child is in utero or breastfeeding, the flu shot causes significant mercury exposure to the baby.

Vaccines and what they contain now, including synergistic impact

Until very recently, vaccinations were the major source of mercury toxicity in children. As of 1999, mercury began to be removed from childhood vaccinations (except the flu shot which is given to children and pregnant women and often still contains a large amount of mercury). However, these mercury-containing vaccines were not recalled—they were just replaced on a volunteer basis by the pharmaceutical companies. Therefore it took until around 2002 or 2003 for a majority of them to be off the shelves.

While fortunately the mercury has been reduced greatly, most vaccinations still contain "trace amounts." This is deceiving because "trace amounts" are still about 3 mcg of mercury per shot. If the safe limit is .1 mcg per kilogram of body weight, the limit for a 5-kilogram baby is .5 micrograms. For infants or children who often receive several vaccines per visit, this can still be a very dangerous amount of mercury and other additives.

In addition to the "trace" amounts of mercury still present, most vaccines also contain, aluminum, formaldehyde, or other substances that are known to be toxic, especially to the brain. The combination of mercury and aluminum (even in small amounts) is far more toxic than just one heavy metal. Cadmium (from smoking), lead, zinc and other heavy metals enhance mercury toxicity. This is a well-known phenomenon in toxicology and was reported many years ago in a 1978 study. It was shown that when the lethal dose of mercury that would kill one out of 100 mice, was combined with the lethal dose of lead that killed one out of 100 mice, the number of mice that died was not two, but all 100. If the toxicity were simple additive, only one or two rats of 100 should have died. Instead, all 100 died (Schubert, 1978). A 2006 study by Bishayi et al. supports this finding and reported "a definite synergistic trend of immunotoxicity during simultaneous exposure to arsenic and lead, that is, a multimetal challenge, as compared to the effects of independent exposure to them" (Bishayi, 2006). The synergistic effect between toxins is important because even though the mercury has been reduced in vaccines, the combined effects of two or more toxins can be much more damaging. Serious testing needs to be done before we assume vaccines with "trace amounts" of mercury are safe.

Other Heavy Metals

Other toxic metals that are high in many children on the autism spectrum are lead, aluminum, antimony, cadmium, bismuth, and even, much more rarely, manganese in high doses (a nutritive metal, necessary at very low levels). Part of this toxicity is due to poor detoxification and low nutrient reserves (which help to push out heavy metals). However, it is a fact that our exposure to toxic metals is higher than ever before in history, and coupled with our exposure to other toxins, it is little wonder that the detoxification systems of many people are overwhelmed.

Dr. Cohen found that mean blood concentrations of lead (another heavy metal) were notably higher in children with autism. The study showed that these children had significantly higher levels of lead than their "normal" siblings (Cohen, 1976:47). Additionally in the study, 44% of the psychotic children (autistic and not autistic), had blood lead levels greater than two standard deviations above the control group (the siblings), supporting that toxins may affect or cause psychiatric conditions. These studies both show decreased ability for those with autism to detoxify heavy metals.

Minimizing exposure to toxins is a crucial step in regaining health. In order to make this step, one must understand all of the possible sources. Here are a few common toxins that should be avoided:

- Lead is commonly found in our environment, in the paint of old homes, in the water supply from old pipes, and in dirt. While the United States government has known for a long time and warned consumers of the dangers of lead's harmful effects on the brain of developing children, it's amazing that there have been so many children's products in the news that have been found to contain lead. Painted toys, vinyl lunch boxes, bibs, and other products from China have been recently found to contain unacceptable levels of lead.

- Aluminum is found as a preservative in vaccinations (as well as the previously discussed mercury). Aluminum is also found in cookware, some canned food, and antiperspirants. A 2007 study sums up the current thinking on Alzheimer's and aluminum (and the damaging effects of aluminum on the brain): "while a direct causal role for aluminum" (and other metals) in Alzheimer's "has not yet been definitively demonstrated, epidemiological evidence suggests that elevated levels of these metals in the brain may be linked to the development or progression of " Alzheimer's (Shcherbatykh, 2007).

- Antimony is in flame retardant used in baby sleepwear and bedding. It is also in carpets and cloth furniture, like couches. Antimony can be quite harmful even at low levels. Antimony is a suspected carcinogen. According to the Ohio EPA's website, "animals that breathed very low levels of antimony had eye irritation, hair loss, lung damage and heart problems. Problems with fertility were also noted." They also state "antimony usage and pollution should be reduced wherever possible." (Ohio EPA, 2002). Additionally, we don't know how toxic the synergistic effects of antimony when it is combined with other heavy metals. Moreover, this is one more toxin to add to the overwhelming burden on the detoxification system.

- Manganese is a nutritive metal like zinc and copper, but in high doses is toxic. Manganese has the effect of lowering serotonin and dopamine levels, and can cause mood disturbances, aggression, and poor impulse control. Golub et al, found that the excess manganese in soy formula "may influence brain development" and have possible "neurobehavioral effects" in rhesus monkeys. (Golub, 2005). A Canadian study concluded that soy or rice beverages "should not be fed to infants because they are nutritionally inadequate and contain manganese at levels which may present an increased risk of adverse neurological effects if used as a sole source of nutrition." (Cockell, 2004). Calcium deficiency increases the absorption of manganese. While manganese won't harm a well-nourished individual, it has the ability to create toxicity in an undernourished child.

Environmental Toxins

Whether environmental toxins are an underlying cause of autism which can change the biochemistry of the system (as it has been proven that mercury can) or they simply exacerbate an overloaded system is not yet thoroughly tested. Mark Schauss, Ph.D., of Carbon Based Labs (www.carbonbased.com) has done extensive research in this area. What is known is that environmental toxins such as xylene, toluene, phthalates (plasticizers), pesticides, and PCBs definitely overburden a taxed liver, kidneys, and many other detoxification routes and can cause seizures and many other physical manifestations. These chemicals affect the entire endocrine system including the thyroid (a problem in many ASD children), adrenals, testes, and ovaries. These potent neurotoxins and pesticides are what appeared to cause serious seizures in Schauss' daughter, which are common in ASD (though she does not have autism). Additionally, phthalates impact boys at a ratio of 4 to 1 compared to girls and Schauss believes these environmental toxins may be the missing link to the rate at which boys are being impacted by autism, as the proliferation of these chemicals corresponds to the timeframe of the rise in autism. When phthalates were first in production in the 1960's only 3% of the people tested positive to them, now 97% of us do. It's certainly possible that the bioaccumulation in the environment and in mothers could account for this rise in autism. Given what we know so far regarding the health of ASD children, Schauss' analogy is apt, "mercury may well 'pull the trigger for autism,' but it is the environmental toxins that 'load the gun'" (Schauss, 2006)

Vaccinations and Immune Function

We find much dysfunction with the immune systems of those with ASD including high rates of ear infections, frequent viral and bacterial infections, high autoimmune markers, elevated levels of pathogenic microorganisms including yeast, and an inability to properly process vaccinations. Autoimmune disorders run in families with ASD. Two of the causes of this poor immune function include mercury (which damages Th1 lymphocytes) and very low nutrient levels.

Infants receive antibodies against infection from the mother through the placenta, and through breast milk. The idea behind vaccines was that after this initial immunity wears off, vaccinations could provide similar protection. In theory, vaccines give an individual controlled exposure to a virus or bacteria in a weakened or killed form, in order for the body to build up antibodies and build immunity toward the germ.

It is commonly accepted that vaccinations have been effective in reducing the prevalence of diseases. While some people credit vaccinations for reducing prevalence of communicable diseases in our society, some believe that communicable disease began to decrease naturally before vaccinations came about. In England and Wales, Kalokerinos and Dettman spoke out against vaccinations in Britain by pointing out that scarlet fever, diphtheria, whooping cough and measles declined 90% from 1850 to 1940, yet widespread vaccinations were not conducted until 1940 (Young, 1999). Some people feel that vaccinations are not the reason for the decline in childhood illnesses.

Outbreaks in vaccinated populations in the recent past show us that vaccinations don't necessarily provide immunity or life-long immunity—and needs to be balanced with the risk of harm to other children (those susceptible to ASD). Additionally, there is the concern that while they may help save some lives, how many are harmed due to complications or lost quality of life from chronic disease? Are we swapping one illness (acute infection) for another illness (chronic inflammatory conditions)? We vaccinate children today more than ever before, and we have more chronic disease in our children. There are entire books dealing with these subjects. Stephanie Cave's book *What Your Doctor May Not Tell You About Children's Vaccinations* is a good place to start.

Vaccinations can cause problems for children with autism in several different ways. As noted earlier, the mercury and aluminum contained in vaccinations is a possible causal factor in the development of autism. Additionally, the virus contained in the vaccines can be a problem. By injecting viruses and foreign particles into the blood stream and artificially activating the immune system while bypassing certain natural first line defenses, adverse effects can result. These dangers typically come from one of three areas (Cave 2001, 22):

1. *Toxins* released by the virus or bacteria can cross into the blood stream and reach the brain. This can cause neurological problems including autism.
2. *Autoimmune reactions*. The body, in some cases, is stimulated to attack other tissue that is similar to the vaccine. This autoimmune reaction—where the body sees itself as foreign and attacks itself—can be caused by measles, tetanus, and flu vaccines.
3. *Infections* can be caused by vaccinations that are supposed to prevent the disease. This can be a full-blown outbreak such as in the case of polio, or a chronic low-grade infection such as from measles.

Medical authorities provide a one size fits all approach for most vaccinations. Take for example, the MMR; while a majority of children have sufficient titers after the first vaccination, common practice it to vaccinate every child with one or two boosters, instead of testing titer levels.

In providing this information, I am not suggesting that all vaccines are harmful or that they should not be given under any circumstance. Vaccine programs supposedly work by "herd immunity" and government experts are always worried about a high enough percentage of vaccine uptake in the community at large. In this, they ignore the individual. Rather, I am suggesting the "radical" notion of questioning authority, studying the efficacy of vaccines, and making a decision based on the best interests of the individual, as well as society as a whole. Appendix III has some suggestions by physicians on potential ways to make vaccinations safer for your child with ASD and the rest of your family.

MMR (Measles, Mumps, Rubella) Vaccination

The MMR vaccine contains three live viruses that are injected into the blood stream. Normally our immune system has several defenses before the virus enters the blood stream. Many parents say that their child's autistic symptoms started after receiving the MMR vaccine. There is much debate in the media on this subject right now, with the government organizations like the CDC (Center for Disease Control) and the medical industry dismissing any connection between the MMR and ASD. A good number of parents I work with did not notice or feel that the onset of autism could be directly correlated with vaccinations; however, the ones who do, make me take notice. The stories are heartwrenching and often similar—a typically developing child receives a vaccination and often has a reaction. If there are more vaccinations, perhaps the next time the reaction is stronger and cannot be denied, but by this time is too late. The child often develops a fever, is sick for days, and never fully recovers. Many parents have sat in my office with tears in their eyes while telling me their experience. I cannot ignore this evidence; it is unconscionable to do so. Additionally, I wonder if other parents just did not notice the connection with the vaccination at the time, as not all reactions are extreme, or even immediate.

Measles

In spite of what people may be lead to believe by the mainstream media and government agencies, there is good evidence to support parental claims that the MMR played a role in their children's regression into autism. Dr. Andrew Wakefield, a pediatric gastroenterologist originally from London, now in the United States, has done extensive research—thirteen studies to date—on autism and the vaccine strain measles virus. While studying inflammatory bowel disorders in children, Wakefield, et al. found eight out of twelve normal children developed autistic symptoms and severe gastrointestinal problems soon after receiving the MMR vaccine (Cave, 2001: 93). In a study Wakefield published in 2002, 75 of 91 children (82%) with developmental disorders and ileal lymphonodular hyperplasia and enterocolitis tested positive for measles virus in their intestinal tissue, compared with five of 70 in the control group. According to Wakefield, "the data confirm an association between the presence of measles virus and gut pathology in children with developmental disorder" (Wakefield, 2002:84). Wakefield and others performed a study in which they studied eight patients with Crohn's disease, three with ulcerative colitis, and nine with autism. Of the nine with autism, they found that three of the children had measles virus in their intestinal tract. All three cases were consistent with the vaccine strain (Wakefield, 2000:727). Of the control group, all cases were negative to any measles virus in the intestinal tract. In another study done by Wakefield, 24 of 25 children with autism had traces of measles in the bloodstream; only one out of 15 children without autism had the virus (Cave, 2001: 66).

Although Wakefield's work has created controversy, he is a very articulate man presenting significant evidence of his findings. His work has also been verified by Dublin professor and pathologist John O'Leary who found measles virus in 96% of children with autism and gave testimony of such findings at a US Congress Committee on Government Reform in 2000. Additionally, in Japan, Kawashima, et al. found:

"The sequences obtained from the patients with Crohn's disease shared the characteristics with wild-strain virus. The sequences obtained from the patients with ulcerative colitis and children with autism were consistent with being vaccine strains. The results were concordant with the exposure history of the patients. Persistence of measles virus was confirmed in PBMC (blood cells) in some patients with chronic intestinal inflammation" (Kawashima, 2000).

In other words, not only did Kawashima, et al. find measles virus as Wakefield did, they were able to verify that it was the vaccine strain virus. Moreover, it was found by Wakefield that virus-infected monocytes traveled to the brain and secrete cytokines toxic to the brain.

The toxic preservatives in vaccines such as mercury weaken the immune system—most particularly by inhibiting the Th1 lymphocytes (a type of white blood cell) from fighting viruses, parasites, and other invaders (Cave, 2001:65). It is important to note that the MMR does not contain mercury; this is because it is a live virus vaccine (and the mercury would kill the live measles virus). After the series of previous mercury-containing vaccinations in the first year, the weakened immune system is not able to appropriately respond to the vaccine and make antibodies against it because the body cannot fight these live viruses appropriately. Because of this weakness, measles can go to the intestinal tract where they multiply and cause a persistent low-grade measles infection. Dr. Wakefield believes the infection inflames the intestinal tract causing extensive inflammation, enterocolitis, and leaky gut. This leaky gut then allows food sensitivities to develop. Two of the most common and serious food sensitivities are to casein (a protein found in dairy) and gluten (a protein found in wheat and other grains), as they form morphine-like substances in some individuals called caseomorphin and gluteomorphin. These morphine-like chemicals can escape the leaky gut, go to the brain, and fit in the opiate receptors causing altered brain function—the outcome is much as if the child were on opium or morphine all day (more about this in the food sensitivities section).

Poor immune function appears to be a factor as to which children respond poorly to the MMR. Wakefield believes that children with a preexisting immune disorder may be predisposed to harboring the virus in their intestinal tract. When they receive the MMR vaccine, it may stimulate an autoimmune response, which leads to the body attacking itself including the central nervous system (Cave, 2001:66).

Eliminating the low-grade measles infection is a crucial step in reducing the inflammation and damage done to the intestinal tract in these individuals. Some DAN! Doctors use vitamin A, antivirals (prescription or natural), and other immune system boosters. Additionally, healing the gut is important. Gluten and casein often cause serious inflammation and formation of opiates in this situation, eliminating gluten and casein is often very helpful for these children—about 50% of individuals with autism experience some benefit. (DAN! 2002, Woody McGinnis)

Congenital Rubella

In 1971, a study conducted by Stella Chess from the New York University Medical Center noted an unusually high rate of autism among children who had congenital rubella—that is, transmission of the rubella virus from an infected mother to the fetus in the first trimester of pregnancy (Mosby, 2002:416)). Of the 243 who had contracted congenital rubella, 18 had complete or partial infantile autism, that is a rate of 412 per 10,000 versus the average rate in Wisconsin in 1970 of .7 in 10,000 (Chess, 1977:69). The data suggest that the rubella virus was the primary etiologic agent in these cases of autism (Chess, 1977:69). The study concluded that the rubella virus invaded the central nervous system. Of the ten cases of complete autism, three recovered and one improved. The two main observations of the study were: a high rate of autism in the group of children with rubella and an unexpectedly large part of the population recovered relatively quickly (Chess, 1977:79). Chess states that a viral invasion of the central nervous system may produce the severe and complex psychopathology that we identify as childhood autism (Chess, 1977:81).

Additionally, I found it intriguing that one of my clients with Asperger's has a mother who was vaccinated with the rubella vaccine while she was pregnant with him. As we have seen in many cases, exposure to the virus either in the wild or through a vaccine can cause the same devastating results for the child; therefore, it isn't at all implausible to suspect that the rubella vaccination in this case caused autism in the child when in utero.

DTP (Diphtheria, Tetanus, and Pertussis) Vaccination

Between 1940 and 1996, reports were released that the pertussis portion of the combination vaccine was causing brain inflammation and chronic brain damage (Cave, 2001:68). After much lobbying, in 1996 a new vaccine was made available, DTaP, which uses partial rather than whole-cell pertussis bacteria. The DTaP was reported to be a safe alternative.

However, Dr. Mary Megson of the Pediatric and Adolescent Ability Center in Richmond, VA believes that the pertussis organism still causes other problems. Megson suggests that the toxins released by pertussis (in both the DTP and DTaP) insert a G-alpha protein defect into genetically at-risk children— those with a family history of at least one parent with a preexisting G-alpha protein defect (Megson, 2000:1). A G-alpha protein defect is characterized by night blindness and various parathyroid, thyroid, and pituitary gland conditions. The data suggest that the toxin separates the G-alpha protein from the retinoid receptors in the hippocampus (Megson, 2000:1) by depleting the store of vitamin A (Megson, 2000:2). It is suspected that vitamin A may reconnect the retinoid receptors, which are essential for vision, sensory perception, language processing, and attention. Interestingly, popular belief says that the sideways gaze of these children is due to social problems stemming from this "psychological" disorder. However, it is now postulated that this sideways gaze may be due to physical challenges with vision due to the G-alpha protein defect and that looking from the corner of the eye may be their adapted way of trying to focus on an object.

We are now discovering through scientific research that the genetic code is not fixed and can be turned on or off with toxins, emotions, and I'm sure other things we have not discovered yet (R. McCraty, 2003).

31

Aluminum increases fluoride's toxic affect on G-proteins, which is essential for thyroid hormone function. (Strunecká) With all of the exposure to fluoride (water fluoridation, fluoride supplementation, exposure in medication and the environment), fluoride levels are fairly high among children with ASD. Could this relatively high level of thyroid dysfunction be in part caused by fluoride? It's certainly possible.

By repleting stores of Vitamin A from supplementation with cod liver oil, children have improved substantially, particularly in the areas of vision, sensory perception, language processing and attention. (Megson, 2000) .

Vaccinations are not completely without risk. Some families and individuals may be at more risk for damage from vaccines. For Points to Consider for Vaccination, see Appendix III.

Candida Overgrowth

Yeast is a pathogen (an agent that causes disease), but under normal, healthy circumstances, it lives in check with the good bacteria in our intestinal tract. When we take antibiotics to kill pathogenic bacteria, we are not only killing the bad bacteria but the beneficial bacteria in our intestinal tract. Getting rid of the good bacteria will allow the yeast to overgrow. It is then difficult for the beneficial bacteria to repopulate. This can happen with anyone healthy or not, from one or many courses of antibiotics, but appears to affect children with autism more severely. Antibiotics are not the only way for yeast to overgrow, but are often a contributing factor.

While candida does not appear to be a root *cause* of autism, it certainly exacerbates the symptoms and bogs down the biochemical processes. It is very common for children on the autism spectrum to have yeast overgrowth. Yeast produce toxic byproducts that absorb through the intestine into the blood stream. Dr. Bruce Semon has seen a significant correlation with yeast overgrowth and autistic symptoms (Shaw, 1998:161).

Since these children are more susceptible to infection such as ear infections, antibiotics are often frequently prescribed, leading to candidiasis (yeast overgrowth), creating a vicious cycle. Since most of us have taken antibiotics at one point or many, why does candida seem to affect children with autism more often? Dr. William Shaw thinks that the weakened immune system is not able to build antibodies against the yeast to mark them as invaders and attack them (Shaw, 1998:28). Another theory of his states that antibiotics allow yeast to overgrow while the immune system is still developing—the immune system does not see the yeast as a pathogen and thus does not develop antibodies to allow the immune system to keep them in check (Shaw, 1998:45). Additionally, once this cycle of antibiotics begins, lack of good bacteria offers no competition for the bad bacteria leading to more bacterial infections and further need for antibiotics.

Yeast negatively affects many functions. Yeast can damage the immune system as described above. They can also disrupt the digestive enzymes. Without the proper digestive enzymes and intestinal wall integrity, nutrients will not be absorbed. Yeast can cause leaky gut and contribute to food sensitivities and opiate exposure in the brain from wheat and dairy as well as other effects described in food sensitivities below. The yeast can produce analogs of the Krebs cycles (energy production cycle) that inhibit energy production.

Dr. William Shaw, Ph.D., a biochemist and founder of The Great Plains Laboratory, states that elevated levels of candida—often referred to as yeast—and its byproducts are common in children with autism (Shaw, 1998:66). The toxins given off by yeast cause autistic symptoms to worsen (Shaw, 1998:161). Toxic metabolites (byproducts from metabolism) from dysbiosis (overgrowth of harmful microorganisms) such as alcohol and formaldehyde, negatively affect the gut and brain (Lang, 2000:4).

UC Irvine research has shown that most children with autism have substantial immune abnormalities of some type, which explains why infections (including candida infections) are so common with children with autism (Shaw, 1998:96). There are many different reasons and theories why the immune system is weakened and why these children seem to get more infections than most. As noted earlier, mercury can weaken the immune system, and/or methylation can be a factor. It is also possible that the yeast itself weakens the immune system, through toxins they give off called gliotoxins. These gliotoxins selectively fragment the DNA of white blood cells (called T-lymphocytes) and macrophages so that they are ineffective in fighting infection (Shaw, 1998:105). Additionally, the gliotoxins affect the sulfhydryl group (or thiol, a sulfur atom with a hydrogen atom) of proteins by inactivating them (Shaw, 1998:105). This information may be an interesting connection to faulty sulfation.

Symptoms of yeast overgrowth include:
- Gas.
- Bloated belly.
- Constipation or diarrhea.
- Hyperactivity.
- Yeast infections (vaginal, nail fungus, athlete's foot, or thrush).
- Itchiness in warm moist areas such as elbows, knees, or genitals.
- Spacey, brain fog, poor memory.
- Chronic nasal congestion.
- Irritability or restlessness.
- Inappropriate laughter.
- Appearing drunk.
- Craving for sweets and fruits.

Many of these symptoms can also be signs of other imbalances such as food sensitivities, but two of the most obvious in my practice have been any type of yeast infection and "strange behavior." I have worked with parents whose children would laugh out of the blue like a "mad scientist" or stumble around the house bumping into things like they were drunk and they are—on yeast toxins.

Regarding testing for yeast, according to Shaw of Great Plains Laboratories, Candida produces an abnormal sugar derivative that is converted to arabinose. Arabinose may alter the function of critical proteins by forming pentosidines. These pentosidines are implicated in the formation of neurofibrillary

33

tangles. Interestingly, these neurofibrillary tangles were also observed by Haley from damage done by mercury to brain tubulin in Alzheimer's disease and autism (DAN! Syllabus, 2002:208),. The neurofibrillary tangles destroy brain-cell function and alter brain structure, likely causing some of the cognitive impairment we often see with autism.

Types of tests for yeast include urinary organic acid tests (OAT), comprehensive digestive stool analysis and/or a blood test for candida antibodies. Great Plains Laboratory says the organic acid marker that indicates yeast overgrowth is arabinose, while Metametrix Lab feels it is arabinitol. While the disagreement continues between the labs, if you suspect yeast overgrowth but you don't see evidence of it in testing, you may want to try various testing methods. I have seen many clients where a yeast overgrowth won't appear on a stool test but will appear on one of the organic acid tests. Testing for candida can be useful; however, sometimes the information is unreliable and the only way to really "test" for yeast is to try a yeast diet and protocol (anti-yeast supplements, probiotics, cultured foods, or medications) and see if the child responds positively.

For children with digestive issues, smelly gas and stool, a history of antibiotic use, or any of the common yeast symptoms, it's a good idea to try a yeast diet and protocol and see how the child responds. When anti-yeast therapy is done, many children improve—some dramatically (Shaw, 1998:161). Often parents are pleasantly surprised with the results. See Appendix IV for a basic yeast diet and explanation of how to rid the body of candida through diet and supplements, and step #9 "Cleaning up the Gut."

Ear Infections/Antibiotics

One of the most common causes of yeast overgrowth is antibiotic use from recurrent ear infections. With a tendency toward poor immune function, infections are more common with ASD. Additionally, clinician and acupuncturist Jake Paul Fratkin feels that antibiotics are often the cause of ear infections. Fratkin says, "Children who use antibiotics have a higher incidence of a repeat infection within six weeks then those who don't use antibiotics. In my own clinical practice, it is obvious that children who never take antibiotics rarely get ear infections." One of the pediatric offices in my area does not use antibiotics as a first round of treatment and they rarely (if ever) have children in their practice with recurrent ear infections. Those children who came from other doctors with chronic infections find their ear infections are greatly reduced when antibiotics are not the primary treatment.

Additionally, many ear infections are due to viruses, and antibiotics will not help those at all. It is important to find ways other than antibiotics to kill bacteria as well as relieve the pain associated with ear infections. Once you realize the negative affects of antibiotics (while they are sometimes necessary), you can begin to search out alternatives that are available (such as mullein and garlic oil). They can often reduce pain and help heal the infection well.

Food Sensitivities

A food sensitivity is similar to a food allergy—although with a delayed response. A food sensitivity is an IgG antibody reaction, versus an IgE reaction associated with food allergy. A food sensitivity is different than a food allergy (IgE), which can create anything from hives to anaphylactic shock. An inability to process a food (food sensitivity) can lead to inflammation, gut injury, and the production of neurotransmitters such as opiates.

A food sensitivity can be inherited from the mother; or, far more likely, develop from leaky gut, which may be a result of yeast overgrowth. When a yeast overgrowth is present, it creates inflammation and damage to the GI tract and can cause food proteins to not be thoroughly broken down, and then "leak" into the blood stream. Our body utilizes the amino acids from proteins, but when the proteins are in the blood stream, they can not be utilized and the immune system reacts against them thinking they are foreign invaders.

Wheat and dairy are the most destructive food sensitivities in autism, as the proteins can turn into opiate compounds. If a protein is not broken down properly into amino acids (possibly due to decreased digestive enzymes), it will form long-chain peptides. It is postulated by Reichelt that these opiates in the urine of individuals with autism "may be due to a genetically based peptidase deficiency in at least two or more peptidases and, or of peptidase regulating proteins made manifest by a dietary overload of exorphin precursors such as by increased gut uptake' (Reichelt, 2003). Without the proper enzymes, gluten from wheat turns into gluteomorphin (Shaw, 1998:126) or gliadinomorphin (Shaw, 1998:202) with gliadin being a fraction of gluten protein. Casein from dairy turns into caseomorphin, also an opiate (Shaw, 1998:202). Gluten is also contained in other grains such as rye, kamut, barley, and oats. These peptides can leak into the blood stream (through leaky gut) and cross the blood brain barrier. These opioid peptides fit into the opiate receptors and function like morphine causing serious neurological problems (Shaw, 1998:202). Many of the symptoms of morphine use are similar to the symptoms we see in autism, such as insensitivity to pain and foggy thinking. Some feel that this is why some children engage in head banging activity; they are so numbed all the time that they are trying to feel something and release the "fog" they're experiencing. Taurine, a sulfur-bearing substance, may have an anti-opiate effect according to Braverman (Braverman, 1987).

In addition to gluten grains and dairy, the other most common food sensitivities include soy, corn, eggs, sugar, chocolate, peanuts, and citrus; however, one can have sensitivities to any foods. I have had clients with sensitivities to peas (a relative of the peanut), beans, and tree nuts. I even see rice sensitivity more often than one would expect. Although these substances that cause food sensitivities do not become opiates, they can have an opiate-like effect in susceptible people, through the creation of exorphins (opioid peptides derived from food sources). Exorphins and endorphins have been shown to have a role in autism (Pizzorno, 2006; Reichelt, 2003)). Food sensitivities can cause behavioral and emotional reactions such as hyperactivity, restlessness, irritability, aggression, temper tantrums, depression, fatigue, being withdrawn, and physical symptoms including constipation, diarrhea, muscle aches, and many more (Rapp, 1991:195). These are some of the symptoms we see with autism, and while food sensitivities are not the cause of autism, identifying and addressing them can reduce many symptoms and assist in behavior and learning.

Food sensitivities can also cause additional physical problems such as inflammation of the intestinal tract or leaky gut. This domino effect could lead to further sensitivities by developing a poor intestinal environment that allows for yeast and other pathogenic organisms to grow and produce toxins that tax the liver and nutrient reserves. Inflammation can result in poor absorption of nutrients affecting any systems of the body including cellular energy, tissue repair, and immune function. Hyperimmune response, also resulting from leaky gut, can cause inhalant and chemical allergies or sensitivities, weakening of the immune system, and possible autoimmune reactions. The effects of food sensitivities can be far reaching.

There are two main ways to test for food sensitivities—through dietary assessment and lab assessment. For dietary testing, there are two common approaches, the implementation of a gluten- and casein-free diet (regardless of lab results), and an elimination/provocation diet that is often used to test many foods, including gluten and casein. A gluten- and casein-free diet is fairly straightforward: it requires the removal of all gluten- and casein-containing foods. It is discussed in more detail in Appendix V. To implement an elimination/provocation diet, the individual removes all common and suspected food sensitivities (including gluten and casein) at once and notices any positive response. Next, every few days, one food is added back—this is the provocation part—identifying any negative reaction (such as headaches, diarrhea, constipation, etc.). Any reaction of this sort can help to identify food sensitivities.

Food antibody assessments are another way to detect food sensitivities and can test 100+ foods quickly and relatively easily. Some parents prefer this to a food elimination diet as the diet can be very challenging for a picky eater to eliminate so many foods from their diet during the testing phase. However, antibody testing does require a blood draw (which is traumatic for some) and has a 10-15% false negative/positive rate. Antibody testing can be a good place to start, but the child's reaction to a food is the best "lab" test.

The dietary intervention for food sensitivities is very individualized. While many children do extremely well on a gluten- and casein-free diet, it is not the solution for everyone. Some children need to have corn and other food sensitivities removed from the diet. Others appear not to have a problem with gluten or casein. Finding the right answer often requires a lot of patience to determine which foods a child is reacting to and how to eliminate them; however, when the right combination is identified the results can be dramatic.

Methylation, Transsulfuration, and Sulfation

The biochemistry of methylation, transsulfuration and sulfation may seem very complex, especially for people who may have been more than a bit relieved to say goodbye to things like calculus when they left high school—but don't be intimidated by it. By getting a grasp of the basics, you will be better able to make decisions for your child. And getting a grasp of the basics simply means getting a good explanation given to you.

One of the reasons we spend so much time studying methylation, transsulfuration, and sulfation is that they explain so much of autism spectrum disorders. These impaired biochemical processes provide a framework that appears to create a detailed picture of much of what ails those with ASD. These pathways are crucial to the health of all humans and when not working properly affect the health and cellular function of many people and conditions (as discussed earlier with Waring's work). Autism is one disorder that is very impacted by these processes. The processes which are reliant on proper methylation, transsulfuration, and sulfation include: detoxification, heavy metal elimination, digestion, immune function, cellular/metabolic function, gut integrity, and microbial balance. (See Figure 2.)

Understanding the basics can help us piece together what systems are not functioning well, why this may be happening, and how to support them to improve function. We can begin to troubleshoot and address why certain reactions may be occurring and which supplements to add. In addition to adding nutrients that are vital to these biochemical cascades, we also want to address and remove toxins that overburden the systems, such as offending foods, environmental chemicals, and microorganisms that give off toxins.

I've created charts that help illustrate the biochemical discussion:
- Figure 2 is an explanation of the methylation, transsulfuration, and sulfation pathways and what the processes are for a functioning system.
- Figure 3 shows how these biochemical pathways (methylation, transsulfuration and sulfation) are typically imbalanced in autism and what the effects are.
- Figure 4 (Nutrients Required) shows some of the nutrients and cofactors ("helper molecules") required on a detailed level to illustrate how complex and interdependent these pathways are.

Here are a few definitions and a reference to Figure 2.
- **Methylation** involves the movement of methyl groups—one carbon and three hydrogens (CH3). Methylation transfers the CH3 from a methyl donor to another molecule. In Figure 2, the methylation pathway involves the top rectangular section.
- **Transsulfuration** involves the formation of glutathione, cysteine and sulfate. It is a primary part of the detoxification system. The precursors (earlier created substances used for this process) of transsulfuration are provided by methylation. In Figure 2, the lower rectangular section is transsulfuration.
- **Sulfation** involves adding on a sulfate group to a biological molecule. Sulfation can activate or inactivate a wide range of biological compounds. Sulfation is dependent on methylation and transsulfuration, to create the compounds needed for the sulfate. In Figure 2, sulfation is the piece on the lower right.

Figure 2: Methylation, Transsulfuration, and Sulfation Pathways

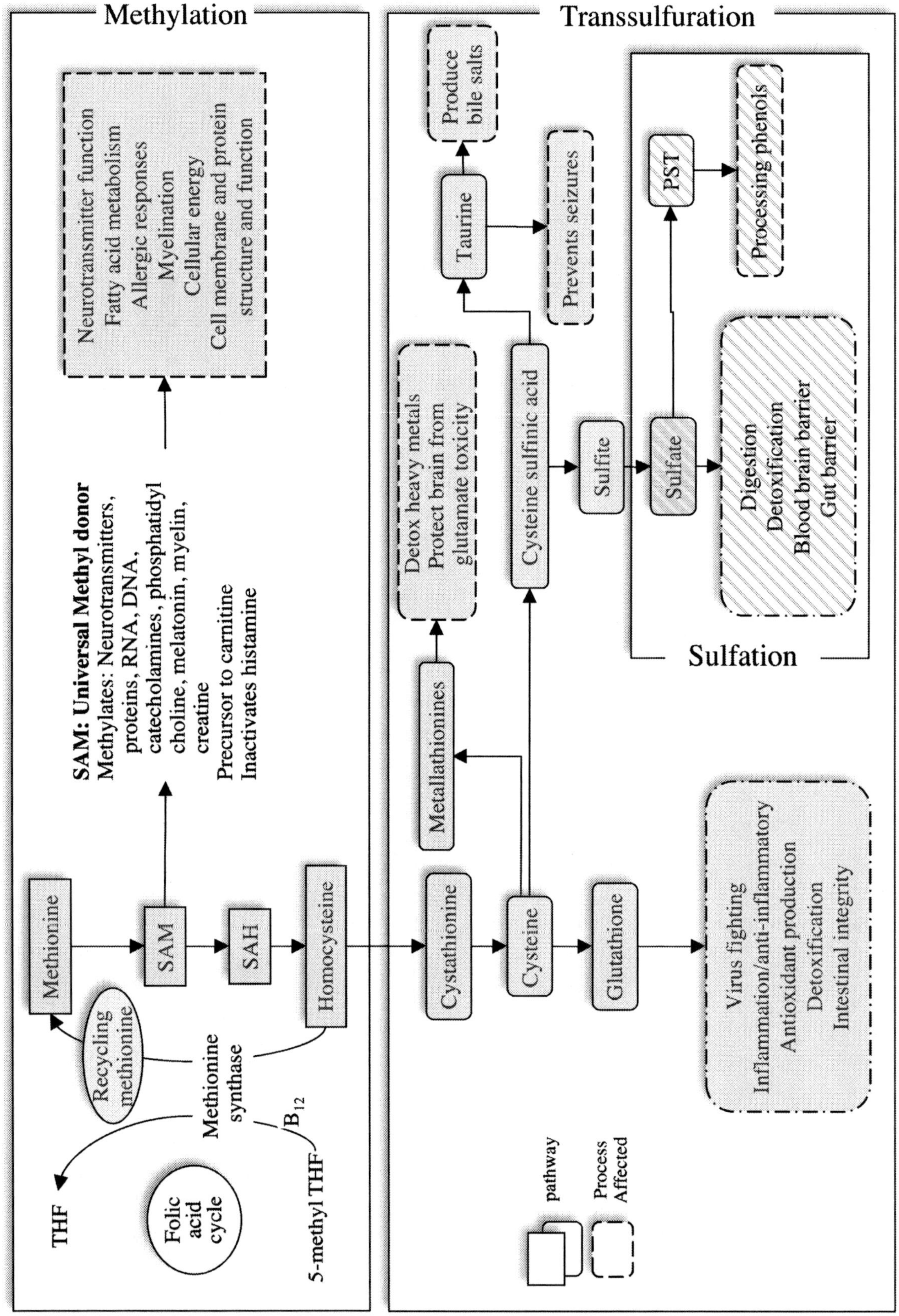

Figure 3: Faulty Sulfation Methylation

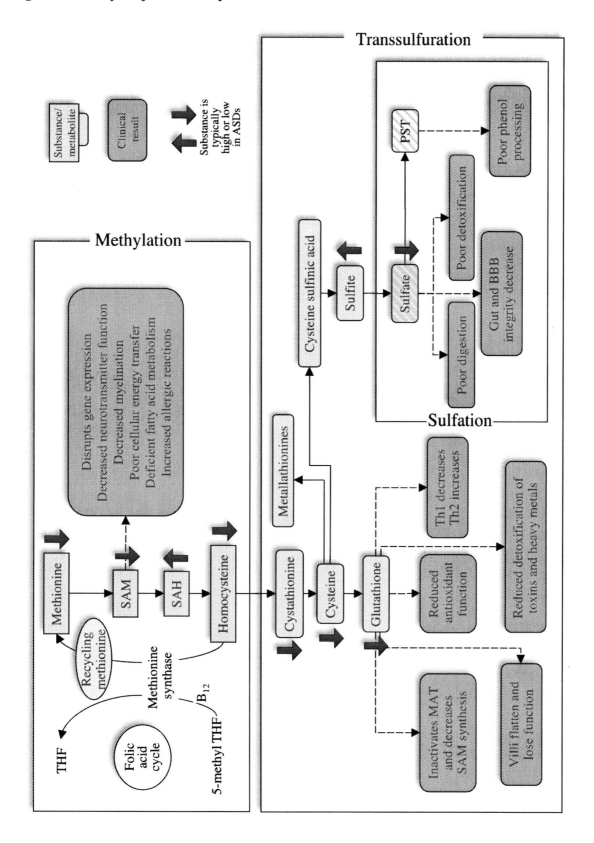

While it is not simple, the biochemical connections of methylation explain so much of the disordered chemistry in ASD that it is worthwhile to get a basic understanding.

Methylation is necessary for health and regeneration. Methylation transfers the methyl group (CH3) from a methyl donor to another molecule. Hence, a methyl donor is simply any substance that can transfer a methyl group (CH3) to another substance. Methylation is vital to life and one of the most essential processes involving DNA. When DNA is methylated, gene expression of that DNA strand is turned off (and if the methyl group is removed, the gene is turned on). Therefore, methylation controls which genes are active and which are inactive. These methylation patterns are established during early development of the embryo, which allows cells to differentiate and helps stabilize the chromosome structure resulting in fewer mutations (Jepson, 2007). However, there is much that can be done once we understand which systems and pathways might be affected, such as supplementing certain nutrients to bypass known biochemical blockages.

In addition to DNA (and RNA, which translates genetic information), vitamins, hormones, neurotransmitters such as dopamine and serotonin, enzymes, and antibodies all depend on methylation. Methylation plays an important role in mood, energy, well-being, alertness, concentration, and visual clarity. Methylation is known (thanks to the work of Jill James) to be impaired in autism (James 2006).

Let's start at the amino acid methionine (Figure 2). Methionine is either taken into the body in the form of food such as meat, dairy, eggs, fish, and sesame seeds, or it is recycled from homocysteine. The major methyl donor in biochemical reactions is S-adenosylmethionine SAM, (also referred to as SAMe) the activated form of the sulfur-bearing amino acid methionine. After donating a methyl group, SAM is converted to SAH (S-adenosylhomocysteine). SAH then creates homocysteine and adenosine. Homocysteine is key here because homocysteine can be recycled back to methionine or can continue down the pathway to create cysteine, glutathione, and more (part of transsulfuration discussed next).

This "recycling process" creates methionine from homocysteine and a methyl donor. This methyl group typically comes from folic acid (when an enzyme called methionine synthase uses vitamin B12 in the form of methylcobalamin to remove the methyl group to create methionine). Additionally, in a parallel pathway, the methyl donor that converts homocysteine to methionine can be trimethylgylcine (TMG) instead of folic acid. This recycling process (using folate or TMG) requires quite a few nutrients and most of them need to be converted in the body from the food form to the usable, active form. For example, folic acid needs to be converted to folinic acid and must go through many other steps to become 5-methyl tetrahydrofolate. Methylcobalamin, the active form of B12, must be converted from cobalamin into methylcobalamin. These are just two of the nutrients needed for this recycling process to illustrate that the substances are not only NEEDED they must be converted into a usable form, often requiring additional nutrients. This begins to shows the complexity needed to perform methylation and the importance of nutritional status.

Figure 4 shows some of the nutrients required for methylation to function properly.

Figure 4: Nutrients Required for Methylation and Transsulfuration

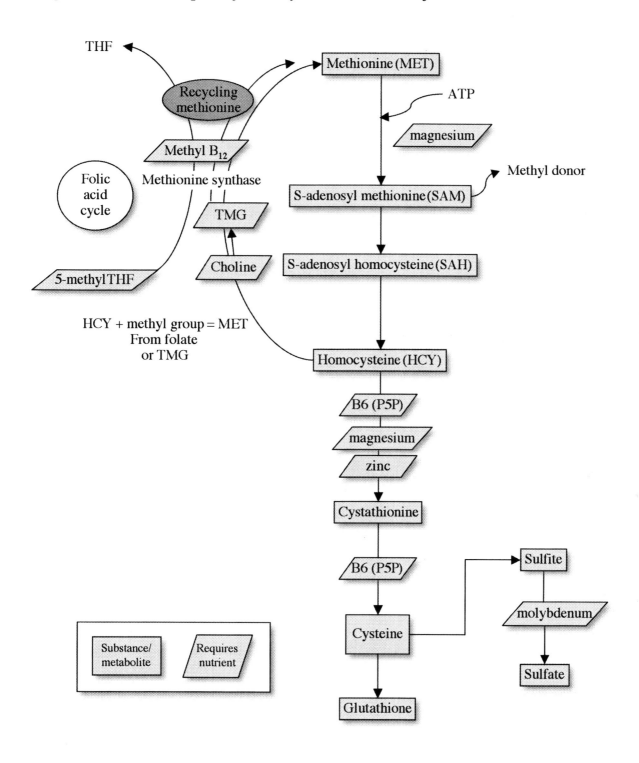

Additionally, if there is oxidative stress, the body will bypass recycling and send homocysteine down to make the antioxidant glutathione (reducing the supply further). This process is explained in more detail below, but it is important to understand that if high levels of oxidative stress are present—and this is very common in children with ASD—the recycling process does not happen because the body believes a more important task must be accomplished.

When you cannot absorb or utilize B12, methylation will be impaired. Children often respond very well to B12 supplementation (typically methylcobalamin injections) with 62% of parents at ARI responding positively (See Appendix VI). James et al. in 2004 and 2006 studies determined that many children with autism live with abnormal metabolic profiles (specifically the transsulfuration pathway discussed later in this chapter). This abnormality creates an increased need for supplemental B12 for the methionine cycle. Boosting this pathway can provide improvement in many cases (James, 2004, James, 2006, Geier, 2006).

As we see the importance of methylation and methyl donors, the use by clinicians of active forms of B12, folic acid, and methyl donors makes sense. Dr. James Neubrander, board certified in Environmental Medicine and a pioneer in methylcobalamin injections for children on the spectrum, has been using methylcobalamin with great results. He has stated that 85 to 90% of children respond positively to the methylcobalamin (not always without some initial side effects). (Arranga 2005) Dr. James' research using supplementation with folinic acid (a folic acid derivative which aids levels of 5-methyl THF) and TMG (trimethylglycine or betaine) that feeds methyl groups to the folate pathway has also showed exciting and promising results. Figure 4 shows some of the nutrients required for these pathways to function.

One problem seen in the methylation cycle of children with ASD, according to Dr. Richard Deth, a professor of pharmacology at Northeastern University in Boston Massachusetts, is that high levels of SAH inhibit methylation (DAN syllabus 2006). Jill James found that in a subset of those with autism, SAH was high while SAM and other transsulfuration markers were low (James 2004).

Furthermore, mercury, thimerosal, and other neurodevelopmental toxins have been found to impair methionine synthase function. (Waly 2004) These toxins are harmful in so many ways to these children and their developing system.

When methylation is not functioning properly, one of the processes that is not properly activated is the large D4 dopamine receptor essential for attention. In a dopamine study researchers found D2 dopamine receptor gene are important in 'reward deficiency syndrome' such as ADHD (Blum 1996). According to Kenneth Bock, M.D., who works with childhood disorders such as autism, one of the malfunctions with dopamine due to insufficient methylation—contributing to ADHD (Bock 2007). This is another example of how an insufficient process can have significant effects on brain chemicals and processing, and in this case is an important explanation for ADHD and the inattentiveness in ASD. I find it fascinating how all of the pieces of the puzzle fit together once you understand the biochemistry and connections.

Transsulfuration

Transsulfuration involves the steps on the biochemical cascade after homocysteine, and deals with substances such as cysteine, taurine, sulfate, and glutathione. These substances are highly implicated in detoxification, antioxidant function, and other important processes.

Jill James has done a great deal of research on transsulfuration in autism and Down syndrome. She has found that children with autism "had significantly lower baseline plasma concentrations of methionine, SAM, homocysteine, cystathionine, cysteine, and total glutathione and significantly higher concentrations of SAH, adenosine, and oxidized glutathione" (James, 2004). These results show that children with autism do not only have poor methylation as discussed above (low methionine, low SAM, high SAH, low homocysteine), but also had poor transsulfuration (low homocysteine, low cystathionine, low cysteine, low glutathione). The levels that were high are also indications of problems with the proper function of these pathways –high oxidized glutathione (spent and oxidized) with low reduced glutathione (strong antioxidant) shows high oxidative stress and potential toxicity and poor transsulfuration (one action of transsulfuration being antioxidant function).

Whether the body chooses to recycle homocysteine back to methionine or take homocysteine down the pathway to glutathione depends on an enzyme process called cystathionine beta synthase. This "decision" requires adequate B6 (in the form P5P, pyridoxyl-5-phosphate) and zinc (Figure 4). If the body is in a state of oxidative stress or toxicity, the pathway will go toward transsulfuration and detoxification functions such as glutathione production.

As homocysteine moves down the transsulfuration pathway (away from methylation), it is converted into cystathionine (which also requires B6 as P5P) to create cysteine. Cysteine can then become one of several things—one of them is taurine, a nutrient that is used to produce bile salts for digestion of fat, and when in short supply can cause seizures. Cysteine can also be used in building metallothioneins (also described earlier in Biochemical Impact of Mercury). This family of proteins is used to detoxify heavy metals, protect the brain from glutamate-induced toxicity, and in gene expression.

Cysteine is also used to create sulfate. This sulfate (or sulfur) is used in a large number of processes called sulfation involving digestion, detoxification, and gut barrier.

Glutathione

When methylation and transsulfuration are working properly, cysteine often continues on to become glutathione. As you will see from Figure 2, methionine is the precursor for cysteine and the rate limiting amino acid for glutathione synthesis (in other words, the rate of glutathione production is limited by how much methionine we have). Because methionine controls how much cysteine and glutathione can be produced, low methionine levels are associated with low cysteine and low glutathione levels. As you can see (Figure 3), we typically find low levels of these precursors and low glutathione.

Glutathione is needed for the antioxidants vitamins C and E to maintain their active form, for proper T helper cells formation and activity, for detoxification of chemicals and heavy metals, and for villi integrity to name just a few of its implications. Low glutathione has a huge negative impact on the health. As you can see from Figure 3, low glutathione causes a reduction in antioxidant production (already low from poor gut absorption and high toxic loads), poor heavy metal detoxification, further decreased intestinal integrity, leaky gut and gut inflammation, Th1 decrease (immune cells that fight infection) and Th2 increase (the cells that increase inflammation and autoimmune conditions).

It is important to note that glutathione's antioxidant potential is lower in males than females, perhaps accounting for part of four to one male to female ratio in ASD (the effects of estrogen and testosterone are possibly other factors as we have discussed in regard to mercury).

Metallothioneins

Metallothioneins (MT) are a family of cysteine-rich proteins with extraordinary metal binding capabilities, which protects the body from the effects of heavy metals. Metallothionein is made from cysteine, part of the transsulfuration pathway.

In a study done by the Health Research Institute and Pfeiffer Treatment Center, 503 ASD patients had very low MT levels—five to eight times less than the control group—in red blood cells (DAN! Syllabus, 2002:182). MT is dependent on zinc and copper, and is induced by toxic metals, physical and emotional stress, and nuclear radiation. MT is the body's primary protection against heavy metals including mercury (DAN! Syllabus, 2002:185). Intestinal MT (MT-IV) provides a barrier in the gut to prevent absorption of toxic metals. MT in the brain and periphery sequesters and neutralizes toxic metals (DAN!, 2002:185). Metallothioneine also impacts immune function, gluten/casein break down, combats inflammation in the gut, and kills candida.

As you can see in the chart on methylation and sulfation (Figure 2), metallothionein requires methylation and transsulfuration (often functioning poorly in those with ASD) for proper manufacturing of these heavy metal detoxifiers. It's plausible to suspect one reason mercury accumulates in these children is due to poor methylation and low metallothionein creating an inability to detoxify mercury—thus allowing it to build up and cause damage. The Health Research Institute and Pfeiffer Treatment Center works extensively with metallothioneins.

Sulfation

Basics and Background on Sulfate and Sulfation

Sulfation involves adding on a sulfate group to a biological molecule. Sulfation is the ability to utilize sulfate in a wide variety of biochemical processes. Sulfation is also the name of a phase II detoxification pathway in the liver that uses sulfate to conjugate (bind to) toxins. For the most part, I will be referring to the first definition. I see the sulfation detoxification pathway as a process within the larger biochemical process of sulfation.

Sulfate is one of the most abundant minerals in the body, or at least it is for most healthy individuals. Sulfate is a combination of sulfur and oxygen molecules. Sulfur, the building block of sulfate, is present in methionine, cystine, cysteine, taurine, glutathione, thiamine, and biotin. Cysteine is used to create

44

sulfate and these other sulfur-containing substances also have a host of important roles in the methylation and transsulfuration pathways.

Sulfate is involved in:
- Enzyme, protein, and tissue synthesis.
- Production of bile acids, digestion, and detoxification.
- Cellular respiration.

As we have learned, cysteine is used to manufacture sulfate. As sulfate is activated by phosphorylation to the active form called phosphoadenosyl phoshosulfate (PAPS), many processes are engaged. Not only is a huge pool of sulfate needed for a large number of enzymes, proteins, and processes, the active form PAPS is needed for detoxification, digestion, and gut/blood brain barrier integrity. For simplicity, although this step is not shown is the diagram, all active sulfate is actually PAPS. Sulfate and sulfation are involved in so many crucial biochemical processes that are often lacking in autism.

Sulfation Function: Research and Clinical Observation

Work done by one of the leading researchers in this field, Dr. Waring, has found that in several studies between 73% and 92% of those with ASD have disordered sulfation chemistry. With such a high percentage of the population affected and the biochemistry fitting neatly into what we see clinically with poor methylation, transsulfuration and sulfation, it is a crucial area to comprehend and that needs more study.

According to a study by Antonino Alberti, Rosemary Waring, and others in 1999, an inability to use sulfate normally to detoxify a sulfur drug like acetaminophen affects up to 92% of low-functioning children with autism (Alberti, 1999:421). Waring and others found that blood plasma levels of sulfate are low in 73% of those with autism. They also found that the activity of platelet phenolsulfotransferase was significantly lower for a small group of children with autism (Waring et al., 1997:40). It appears that faulty sulfation affects a great percentage of those with autism.

In individuals with autism, sulfate is being dumped into the urine (Waring & Klozvra, 2000: 25) regardless of abnormally low plasma sulfate levels (Waring, 1997:42). Since the body appears to be dumping the sulfate that it needs so much, Susan Owens, a cutting-edge researcher on sulfation states that this suggests that something about how sulfate is regulated systemically is not working properly (Owens, 2001:217).

To take this a little deeper, the sulfation process involves the action of many sulfotransferases—that is, sulfate enzymess—including one that processes phenols called phenolsulfotransferase) (Owens, 1998:2). Sulfate must be activated (phosphorylated) before it can be used by sulfotransferases (Owens, 2000:1). This involves the formation of the molecule phosphoadenosyl phophosulfate (PAPS), which is the rate-limiting step in sulfation and affects all sulfotransferases. In a hypothesis put forth by Owens, if the lack of PST activity in autism is caused by the cells lacking sulfate, than all of other sulfotransferase enzymes that use sulfate would be affected as they draw from the same sulfate pool. Therefore, we would clinically see improper functioning of all sulfotransferase activities in autism and indeed we do (Owens, 2000:1). The improper functioning is implicated in:

- Poor detoxification.
- Lack of integrity in the gut. Sulfate joins with saccharides to form the protective layer in the gut called glycosaminoglycans or GAGs (Lang, 2000:1). These GAGs also aid in formation of the blood brain barrier.
- Poor digestion. Gut hormones cholecystokinin (CCK) and gastrin are sulfated by tyrosine protein sulfotransferase (Owens, 2001:1). Refer to the chart on sulfate's role in digestion (Figure 5) to see the cascade of digestive processes that are initiated by CCK and gastrin.
- Peptides and proteins such as IgA, IgG, and C4 are sulfated.
- Altering hormones such as testosterone, estrogen, and DHEA

This primary set of the affects of faulty sulfation leads to a larger set of secondary problems, which perpetuate a vicious cycle of further imbalances. For example:

- Poor detoxification permits exogenous toxins such as mercury from vaccinations, pesticides from produce and meat, additives and preservatives from processed foods to cause further damage to the body or act on the brain as drugs or neurotoxins. Additionally, endogenous sources such as hormones and neurotransmitters, continue to circulate in the body and brain disrupting the endocrine system and negatively affecting brain function and behavior.
- Gut permeability allows partially digested proteins to absorb into the blood stream converting to opiates causing cognitive impairment. Leaky gut also reduces absorption of nutrients essential to cellular function, brain function, and tissue repair, which decrease energy, mood, cognitive function, and gut repair. GAGs used to line the intestinal tract also protect the brain from toxins through the blood brain barrier. This makes the brain "leaky" causing toxins to more easily cross from the blood into the brain causing impairment and/or damage.
- Poor digestion also leads to poor breakdown and absorption, which in turn decreases nutrients needed for proper detoxification, immune function, and neurological function. Poor digestion impairs protein, fat, and carbohydrate breakdown required for the building blocks for neurotransmitters and tissues (protein), essential fatty acids for cognition and cellular function, and carbohydrates for energy.
- Peptides and proteins disrupt the effectiveness of the immune system, allowing pathogens to cause infection in the body. Chronic infections are often present in autism such as ear infections, low grade measles infections in the gut, etc.
- Sex hormones regulate the action of sulfotransferases, which may help explain why almost four times as many boys as girls are diagnosed with autism (Powers, 2000:14).

Causes of Faulty Sulfation

When sulfation is impaired we often refer to it as faulty sulfation.

Faulty sulfation could be caused by so many reasons: any "breaks" along the methylation, transsulfuration, or sulfation cascade could affect sulfation. There are several genes identified with methylation responsibilities, and the cause of faulty sulfation could be genetic (from a parent) or acquired (mercury from vaccinations), or both. Particular genetic factors could lay the groundwork for a sulfation system more easily injury by mercury. It's also possible that if the mercury poisoning is severe enough that this alone could be enough to knock out these biochemical pathways.

Additionally, chlorine seems to negatively affect sulfation. This may be because chlorate is a biological substance that strongly blocks sulfation and the fact that low reserves of sulfate and other nutrients needed to create the enzyme phenolsulfotransferase (PST) may be further wiped out by the need to detoxify the chlorine. High toxic load that uses up detoxifying substances play a part in causing faulty sulfation.

In addition to poorly functioning biochemical pathways, Owens states six places/ways sulfation can be impaired (Owens, 2001:4-9):
1) Lack of raw material.
2) Improper function of enzymes that are needed to generate inorganic sulfate from its precursors.
3) Movement of sulfate across membranes.
4) In the interaction with the purine metabolism involved with converting inorganic sulfate into activated sulfate.
5) In the expression and action of sulfotransferase enzymes.
6) In the recycling or retention of systemic sulfate.

Sulfation and Phenols

In chemistry, a phenol is a phenyl ring or benzene ring (C_6H_5) with a hydroxyl group (-OH). The cell membrane of a phenol is composed of both water and fat. This means it can easily cross the blood brain barrier and get into the brain. Norepinephrine, a neurotransmitter, is a phenolic compound. Plants often create phenolic substance called salicylates. Food additives made from a petroleum base are phenols. Some of these chemical phenols (food additives) look very similar to neurotransmitters and act as neurotoxins by binding to neurotransmitter receptors. From there they artificially stimulate the brain and cause "noise" manifesting as hyperactivity, headaches, aggression, red ears, and many more symptoms (see Appendix VII). Dr. Ben Feingold, pediatrician and allergist at Kaiser Permenente in San Francisco in the 1970's, found that these substances, when the could not be properly processed and detoxified, build up and enter the brain causing disruption (Feingold, 2001).

Phenolsulfotransferase (PST) is an important enzyme that processes sulfur compounds, namely phenols— hence the name phenol-sulfo-tranferase. PST will process phenols such as artificial food ingredients, salicylates (naturally found in fruits and vegetables), and phenolic amines such as dopamine and serotonin. Dr. Feingold recognized that this process was not working correctly in children with ADHD when they were unable to process artificial ingredients and foods high in phenols. In one study Waring conducted, she and her team found along with low levels of plasma sulfate (a building block for PST) in the children with autism, a significantly lower activity of PST in a subgroup of children with autism.

Signs of phenol intolerance or poor processing of phenols are helpful in determining faulty sulfation. These reactions (unlike food intolerances) come on pretty quickly, typically 20 minutes to two hours after consumption. Some of the most common signs include: hyperactivity, fatigue, inappropriate laughter, red cheeks and ears, aggression, self-injurious behavior, impatience, poor sleeping habits, headaches, and poor neuro-muscular function. However, be aware that many of these manifestations can also be signs of other imbalances. Two of the most obvious signs are red cheeks and/or ears and an unusual craving for phenolic/salicylate foods. Some of the more confusing (but common) signs are inappropriate laughter, often seen with yeast overgrowth; self-injurious behavior and aggression, often seen with gluten and casein opiates; and fatigue or hyperactivity, which could be related to many things including yeast overgrowth. As it can be confusing, take all of the signs, symptoms, and reactions into consideration when trying to determine if phenols are an issue, most parents find it very helpful to keep a journal documenting these things. Without some sort of documentation, the detective work necessary may prove impossible.

Diet is very helpful to address a sulfation/phenol issue. We will address this later in detail with the Feingold and Failsafe Diets.

Sulfate and Sulfation in Systems Impaired in Autism

Sulfate and sulfation are so important in so many of the body's systems affected in autism that it is helpful to highlight them individually. One of the things that convinced me first that autism had biochemical underpinnings was seeing how many systems were negatively impacted with faulty sulfation. These systems include:

- Detoxification
- Gut and brain permeability
- Digestion
- Neurodevelopment
- Immune system

I'm not suggesting that sulfation is the only answer behind the autism epidemic; however, it clearly shows that there is a biochemical basis for autism—some pieces known, others still unknown.

Sulfate and Detoxification

In addition to PST, Phase II liver detoxification uses sulfate throughout many detoxification pathways, most significantly during sulfation (sulfate conjugation). The sulfation pathway detoxifies neurotransmitters, steroid hormones, certain drugs, phenolic compounds, toxins from the environment, and toxins from the body such as hormones, neurotransmitters, and intestinal bacteria. According to Pizzorno, "since sulfation is [also] the primary route for the elimination of neurotransmitters, dysfunction in this system may contribute to the development of some neurological disorders" (Pizzorno, 1999:104). I believe this is a significant finding for ASD. Acetaminophen (also known as paracetamol) is a drug detoxified primarily through the sulfation pathway, and therefore often used in studies and lab tests to assess sulfation function. (See Detoxification under the Intervention section for more on Phase I and Phase II liver function.) Sulfation is a key liver detoxification pathway that is often disrupted with ASD (www.gdx.net, 2001:1).

Glutathione conjugation, methylation, and amino acid conjugation are also detoxification pathways in the liver that require sulfate. Therefore when sulfate is low, a great majority of the liver detox processes are not functioning well, causing poor detox and accumulation of toxins—as we see in those with ASD.

With detoxification reduced, other substances such as mercury and yeast toxins can build up in the body as well. All of these exogenous and endogenous chemicals overload the detoxification system further causing damage to the body systems and organs, and greatly impairing cognitive function.

The enzymes required for sulfation are sulfotransferases. When sulfation is working properly, it decreases toxicity and increases water solubility of toxins, allowing the toxins to be excreted in the urine and bile.

Sulfate needed for sulfation comes from cysteine through a several step process called sulfoxidation (Pizzorno, 1999:104). Sulfite oxidase, an enzyme, metabolizes these sulfites into safer sulfates, which are then excreted in the urine (Pizzorno, 1998: 106). In patients with neurological disorders, it appears that this enzyme, sulfite oxidase, responsible for sulfoxidation of cysteine to sulfate is often deficient, leading to elevated plasma cysteine/sulfate ratio (Heafield, 1990:110). Heafield's study shows that some individuals accumulate cysteine and have low sulfate levels (Heafield, 1990:110).

If someone is low in sulfate, as these children typically are, it would seem to make sense to add more sulfur-containing foods and supplements to the diet. However, according to Pizzorno, when the sulfoxidation detoxification pathway isn't working very well, people become sensitive to sulfur-containing drugs and foods containing sulfur or sulfite additives (Pizzorno, 1998:106). Additionally, Lang states that many of these substances (such as cysteine) can cause distress or exacerbate problems (Lang, 2000:4) so it is not as simple as adding cysteine or broccoli (a sulfur-containing food) to the diet.

Sulfate in Gut and Brain Permeability

Glycosaminoglycans (GAGs) are long unbranched polysaccharides that have many functions including intestinal integrity. GAGs need to be sulfated (have sulfate added) in order to work. According to Owens, unsulfated GAGs have one of the greatest impacts on those with autism. As Owens discusses, GAGs are highly varied, specific, and regulated. Furthermore, they influence the following basic cellular processes (Owens, 2001:1):

- Membrane function (gut and brain membrane integrity)
- Protein/protein interactions
- Ligand/receptor interactions
- G protein signaling
- Calcium signaling
- Gap junctions (cell to cell communication)
- Differentiation
- Growth
- Endocytosis
- Management of cations at the cell surface.

According to Owens (2001:3), the GAG processes listed above are threatened when the sulfate pool is too small. In the presence of infection (such as a chronic measles infection) in the gut (Murch, 1993:711) and other infections in the body (Zapata-Sirvent, 1994:1), GAGs are shed. Macrophages then come to the site from which they've been shed, break down the tissue and release the sulfate, after which the sulfate is excreted in the urine. According to Owens, this combination of events in response to infection could provide an explanation of how autistic enterocolitis or chronic ear infections might induce systemic sulfation problems (Owens, 2001:5).

Chronic inflammation of the gut can be caused by many factors and can deplete the body of antioxidants, sulfate-derived glutathione, and methionine (Lang, 2000:4). This inflammation can be caused or exacerbated by the following:

- Insufficient sulfation of GAGs
- Measles infection (naturally occurring or through immunization) (Wakefield, 2000:723)
- Food allergens and intolerances (Shaw, 1998:125), including opiate formation
- Dysbiosis from yeast, or bacteria
- Parasites
- Unneutralized gastric acid (Lang, 2000:4)
- Chronic and excessive autoimmune response
- Incomplete digestion of fats and proteins

In the kidneys, unsulfated GAGs allow the loss of these sulfates. This matches the research as Waring found sulfate to be low in the blood and high in the urine. When sulfate is low and GAGs are unsulfates, may systems malfunction, most especially the gut barrier and the brain barrier—two locations where good defenses are needed.

Sulfate and Digestion

Regarding the role of sulfate in digestion (see Figure 5), sulfate triggers gastrin, which starts a cascade of other reactions for digestion (Lang, 2000:1). Gastrin releases hydrochloric acid (HCl) and pepsin, which increase gastric acidity thereby providing better breakdown and utilization of proteins and amino acids (including the sulfur-bearing amino acids) that are required for building essential tissues, enzymes, neurotransmitters, and hormones. HCl lowers the pH to stimulate secretin. Secretin is a digestive hormone produced in the duodenum and jejunum when partially digested protein enters the intestine. Secretin stimulates the pancreas to produce bicarbonate, bile, and pancreatic enzymes (Mosby, 2002, 1553) for further digestion. Gastrin stimulates the release of cholecystokinin, which activates the release of bile (Lang, 2000:1). As noted earlier, bile is an important component for clearing toxins from the body. Bile emulsifies fats, allowing for further digestion and assimilation by the small intestine (Mosby, 2002: 201). Interference in the flow of bile will result in the presence of unabsorbed fat in the feces and poor assimilation of essential fatty acids. Gastrin also stimulates pancreatic enzyme secretions, which are required for further digestion of fats, carbohydrates, and protein. Clearly, sulfate is crucial in the process of digestion.

Figure 5: Role of Sulfate in Digestion

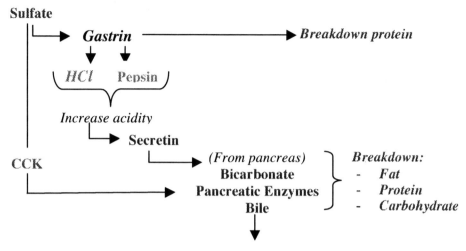

Emulsifies fat /Clears toxins

As you can see, without sulfate, the beginning of the digestive process is impaired. If you do not have enough sulfate to kick off gastrin, you will not have enough HCl to break down your food properly. This in turn may not allow food to be released into the small intestine and instead comes up through the esophagus. I attended a talk given by a popular gastroenterologist at Stanford where he discussed acid reflux in those with ASD. He mentioned that acid blockers are often used to relieve symptoms, but as they did not make the condition better, the patient would have to be on the drug for life and if the drug failed, surgery was the other option. I asked him if it is possible that this poor sulfation could cause low HCl, slow gastric emptying and the acid reflux seen in so many of these children, and whether addressing the biochemistry might alleviate the problem. While I was excited about this hypothesis, the doctor did not respond to my question. If mainstream medicine is not providing relief for acid reflux, there are other schools of thought that may help.

As discerned above, secretin does significantly improve digestion; however, it misses the beginning of the digestive process starting with gastrin. Back in early 2000, secretin was the "hot therapy" to try. While it seemed to help some, it did not prove to the positive intervention clinicians hoped for. Possibly this is because it only helped with part of the process—because gastrin (which was bypassed instead of boosted) is crucial for:

- Initiating the secretion of pepsin. Pepsin, along with HCl, will break down proteins further.
- Stimulating the release of mucous for protecting the submucosal and epithelial lining of stomach and duodenum from inflammation and degradation.
- Stimulating the contractions of the gallbladder to release bile into the duodenum to breakdown fats, fatty acids, and fat-soluble vitamin A.
- Stimulating CCK, which initiates the gallbladder's release of bile salts that clear toxins, and digest fat and fatty acids.
- Simulating release of pancreatic bicarbonate to neutralize acid from stomach.

Sulfate and Neurodevelopment

At birth, humans have most of their neurons formed; however, about 90% of the brain's cells, called glial cells, are only beginning to form at this stage (Owens, 2001:9). As Stringer observed, this process involves highly sulfated heparin sulfate (Owens, 2001:10). Before birth, the mother begins to supply significantly more sulfate to the blood and across the placenta to prepare the infant for this process (Owens, 2001:9). This maturation process of the brain is most intense just before the age of two, just at the same time as a majority of vaccinations are given (Owens, 2001:226).

For mothers with faulty sulfation, they may not supply enough sulfate and the process of neuronal formation may not function optimally. Of additional note on pregnancy, oxytocin is required for delivery. Oxytocin needs sulfate. If a birth is not progressing, perhaps due to a lack of oxytocin, a synthetic form called pitocin is often used. Research indicates that a higher percentage of mothers who give birth to children who become autistic required pitocin during labor. This could indicate a hereditary fault with sulfation. Additionally, oxytocin is the "social hormone" responsible for social recognition and bonding and may account for some cases of social abnormalities in children with ASD (Owens, 2001:9-10).

At the same time as myelination (insulation) of neurons is taking place, other neurons form perineuronal nets. These perineuronal nets require chondroitin sulfate and are abnormal for those with AIDS, dementia, and Rett syndrome, disorders which have similar losses of sulfate as autism. (Owens, 2001:10). According to Owens, these nets are implicated in:

- Modulation to the auditory system
- Motor areas that regulate bilateral, complex, and skilled movement
- Input from the visual areas associated with movement
- Neurons that govern hearing, sound and tones
- Governing posture, spinning
- Localization of sound

According to Owens, the formation of these nets appears to also be dependent on repetitive use of the neuron and may explain why children with ASD prefer repetitive movements (as the neurons can form later, just more slowly). She believes that repetitive therapies like ABA or sensory integration might help with brain development (Owens, 2001:12).

Dr. Boyd Haley's work on mercury poisoning explains the damage done to the brain by mercury through the formation of neurofibillary tangles resulting from the stripping of tubulin in the hippocampus. He refers to the densely packed and undeveloped cells we see with autism and hypothesizes that mercury may stop neuronal growth and account for the undeveloped brain (DAN! 2002). The negative impact of mercury on methylation and sulfation suggests that mercury may affect the brain both directly and indirectly.

Sulfate and Immune Function

If sulfate stores are low and PST is not functioning to clear phenols properly, this can have a strong negative effect on the immune system. For example, there is evidence that strong phenolic substances (such as petroleum-based substances) may drop T-suppressor cells or total T-cell numbers. Phenolic exposure also was found to depress serotonin, and elevate histamine and prostogladins. Phenols can lead to a toxic overload and/or stimulate allergic response.

Phenols burden the detoxification system, wiping out many of the antioxidants needed for immune function like vitamin A, C and E. Additionally glutathione, which is important for Th1 and Th2 ratios, is reduced or wiped out with a high phenol load. Mercury, the same substance that directly depresses immune function also blocks sulfation. There are many direct and indirect responses between sulfation and immune function.

COMMON PHYSIOLOGICAL IMPLICATIONS IN ASD

Liver and Detoxification

Liver function

The liver, our major organ for detoxification, works in two phases. Both Phase I and Phase II pathways must be working correctly for detoxification to occur successfully. Phase I prepares the toxin for final detoxification in Phase II where a substance conjugates (binds) to the toxin to neutralize it. Glutathione is a conjugation substrate (that is, the substance to which the toxin is being bound) used to neutralize Phase I metabolites. Increasing glutathione levels that are low in these children is critical because often their internal mechanism to create glutathione—the methionine pathway—is not working properly. Garlic, dandelion, lysine, aloe, and rice bran extract are food sources that help to increase glutathione levels.

Think of Phase I and Phase II as two pools or funnels that flow into one another, finally leading to a waterfall and dumping into the ocean. The first funnel is Phase I liver detoxification process that uses enzymes (called Cytochrome P450) and the second funnel is Phase II, which binds a substance to the Phase I product neutralizing it. One of the challenges with this system is that a toxic substance is converted to an even more toxic substance at the end of Phase I. If this Phase I substance cannot by neutralized by Phase II, we have a more toxic substance on our hands than we did to begin with. Given the pool or funnel analogy, these highly toxic Phase I metabolites cannot be processed fast enough by Phase II and these toxic intermediaries overflow the funnel and spill into the system.

Detoxification in Autism

The above scenario is what often happens in autism. In those with ASD, Phase II detoxification is typically slow and the "extra toxic" metabolites from Phase I are causing even more damage than they would otherwise. Phase I is overactive, either overactive in comparison to Phase II or genuinely overactive. Ideally, we would increase Phase II function. However, even decreasing Phase I and lowering the rate at which the really toxic metabolites are created helps. Be aware that many children with autism are also low in Phase I so this is often a short-term remedy, not necessarily a solution.

For information on this, and on ways to address detoxification in general, depending on the biochemistry and liver function of the individual, see Part 3, Step #12, *Detoxification*.

Immune System and Inflammation

Immune System

Th is the acronym for T helper cells. T helper cells are a crucial component of the immune system. Th1 is the cellular immune system—the virus/microorganism fighting side of the immune response that kills organisms directly with macrophages. Th2 is the humoral immune system—mediated by antibodies, and is involved with the inflammatory and autoimmune responses. Ideally, the Th1 and Th2 systems are in some sort of balance, each responding appropriately when necessary: fighting viruses and bacteria efficiently, turning on and off the inflammatory response when appropriate.

Inflammation and Immune Function in Autism

However, balance between Th1 and Th2 is often not found in children with ASD. Typically in ASD, Th1 lymphocytes are low and the Th2 arm of the immune response predominates. As a result, children are unable to fight the bacteria causing ear infections, the viruses in the vaccinations, and yeast infections in the gut. They are not able to mount a sufficient response.

Additionally, an inability to kill viruses, bacteria, and yeast can create inflammation in the brain—as with streptococcal bacteria that creates an autoinflammatory response in the brain resulting in a condition called PANDAS. An overactive Th2 response increases antibody and autoimmune problems that are frequent in ASD. It is not uncommon for children on the autism spectrum to have elevated autoantibodies to myelin basic protein, to the thyroid (Hoshimoto's thyroiditis), or to the pancreas (diabetes). The inflammatory response is overactive and the anti-inflammatory response is underactive. This often creates significant inflammation throughout the body including the gut, the brain, or virtually anywhere.

Asthma

According to Bock in his book, *Healing the New Childhood Epidemics*, "Children on the autism spectrum…have higher incidence of asthma. The presence of asthma or allergies during a mother's pregnancy doubles her change of having an autism child. Children with asthma had significantly higher rates of ADHD behaviors" (Bock, 2007:123). He also states, "Asthma, hypothyroidism, and allergies are the three most common co-morbid physical disorders among people with autism" (Bock, 2007:123).

Allergies are behind the inflammation of asthma. Many parents report asthma attacks being triggered by allergies. The immune system reacts to certain foods or chemicals creating inflammation. That inflammation can create inflammation throughout the body, including the lungs. Toxins can exacerbate asthma by creating further inflammation in the body. Feingold Association has found that artificial ingredients—artificial colors and flavors and MSG—are really serious triggers for asthma. Pollution is one of the biggest causes of asthma.

Avoiding chemical and food allergies and sensitivities is very important. Raw milk studies showed lower incidences of allergies and asthma with those children who consumed "farm milk" (raw milk) (Waser, 2006). Magnesium and calcium relax the muscles around the lungs. Cod liver oil with omega-3 and vitamin A is a good supplement for reducing inflammation associated with asthma.

GI Tract and Digestion

Digestive Function in Autism

Digestion is affected in a high percentage of children with autism. According to ARI, 50% of children with ASD have constipation and/or diarrhea (autism.com). Leaky gut and food sensitivities are very common. There are many causes for this. As we saw earlier, fault sulfation can weaken intestinal integrity and digestion, toxins can damage the gut, antibiotic use can contribute to yeast overgrowth and dysbiosis leading to inflammation and gut damage, food sensitivities can contribute to further inflammation, viruses (wild and vaccine) can create ongoing infection and damage to the gut. As these are just *some* of the causes and contributors to poor digestive function and GI health, it is not surprising that digestive issues affect so many children with ASD.

There are many dietary and supplement interventions that can support digestive wellness. Diet has a positive effect on 50-66% of children depending on which diet is implemented. Supplements such as enzymes, probiotics and nutrients to nourish and heal the gut are very useful in healing the gut. Bile salts can help when the gall bladder is sluggish to break down fats. Taurine can help build bile salts. HCl is substance important for digestion (see more below). Diet and supplement ideas are discussed throughout the supplement and diet section in Part II, *Compendium of Nutritional Strategies and Opportunity*.

Constipation

Constipation is one of the most common and problematic digestive disturbances. Firstly, constipation is uncomfortable. It can even be painful. Fear of elimination can exacerbate the constipation and problem. Constipation can encourage growth of dysboitic organisms and decrease colon health. Most importantly, when the stool sits in the colon, toxins in the stool reabsorb through the intestinal wall. When this happens, irritability, stimming, and discomfort can increase. When chronic constipation exists, the colon can stretch making the muscles weak—peristalsis (contraction of the intestinal muscles that move stool) and the urge to have a bowel movement decreases. This creates a cycle of constipation.

Constipation can be addressed through diet and supplementation. Diet reduces inflammation and improves GI health. Opiates in medicine (morphine, codeine) are known to slow motility (movement of the stool through the colon), and opiates from gluten and casein can do the same. Supplements can support regular bowel movements. Vitamin C can help with constipation from two angles: vitamin C can loosen stool and help raise HCl levels (as low levels can contribute to constipation). See Part II, *Compendium of Nutritional Strategies and Opportunity*. Enemas and colon hydrotherapy (not discussed here) can also help stop the cycle of chronic constipation.

Hydrochloric Acid (HCl)

It is common for HCl to be low with children on the spectrum. Counter-intuitively and contrary to what we are commonly told, heartburn is often cause by low HCl, not high. Therefore, decreasing stomach acid with a medication may work in the short run but doing so will make the situation worse in the long run. HCl is also required for proper absorption of minerals such as calcium.

If a child refuses to eat meat, consider that he does not feel well eating it because he may not be able to digest it well. This may be because digestion is not strong enough to breakdown protein due to insufficient HCl. If this is the case, consider addressing HCl production. This can be done in various ways: try HCl capsules, or use bitter foods and herbs like Swedish Bitters to stimulate the vagus nerve to tell the stomach to release HCl. Increasing vitamin C intake, in the form of ascorbic acid, can also increase HCl. Also make sure zinc is at adequate levels, as zinc controls the enzyme that makes HCl.

Stress can be a factor—inhibiting or stimulating HCl release. Addressing the adrenals as needed, will certainly be helpful for many systems. There is more information about addressing adrenal problems in Adrenals in this section.

For those who have truly high acid, a factor to consider is MSG, as ingestion of MSG has been reported to cause excess acid and heartburn. Soothing herbs such as aloe vera, slippery elm, and deglycyrrhinizinated licorice (DGL) can help with high acid.

A doctor can quantifiably measure high or low acid with the Heidelberg test. This test involves a capsule that is swallowed (then pulled up), that measure the stomach acid. Short of that, there is the beet juice test, a simple home-based test (see *Assessements*) that can give you an idea if HCl is low. Finally, the Comprehensive Digestive Stool anaylsis tests show protein breakdown, which is an indirect indicator of HCl status.

Endocrine and Glandular Function

The endocrine system is complex and its many components work together. When one part is imbalanced, other parts are often affected. The thyroid, adrenals, and pancreas are a few of the important organs associated with endocrine function. Endocrine system is an information signaling system that uses chemical messages (hormones) to communicate.

Thyroid

According to ARI, thyroid disorder is higher in autism than the general population. The thyroid regulates metabolism, energy, and body temperature, and low thyroid can cause fatigue, depression, constipation, and irritability—many of the symptoms we see with autism. Low thyroid function is the major cause of mental retardation in the world.

You can test thryoid function in the lab but be aware that ranges can be too broad, and standard tests only test T4 (thyroxine); however, there are labs that test: free T4 and free T3 (triiodothyronine), reverse T3, TSH (thyroid stimulating hormone), and thyroid autoantibodies. It's important to test free T3 early (something not done on standard medical screenings), as the mental retardation associated with low thyroid is not reversible. See *Assessments* in *Impact of Nutrients* section.

Causes of hypothyroid include:
* Deficiencies in nutrients such as iodine, selenium, iron, magnesium, zinc, B6, Vitamins A, C and E. We see these same deficiencies in autism.
* Autoantibodies, common in autism
* Toxic exposures, common in autism
* Too many polyunsaturated fats, common in a Standard American Diet
* Adrenal insufficiency, common in autism

Symptoms of Hypothyroidism:

- Fatigue
- Weight gain, however, children with autism may be thin and undersized
- Dry hair or skin
- Cold intolerance; cold hands, feet or fanny
- Muscle cramps and/or frequent muscle aches
- Constipation or hard stools
- Depression
- Irritability
- Inattentiveness

There are a variety of supplements to support the thyroid including thyroid glandulars, iodine, and other herbal and nutrient formulas. According to ARI, "Synthetic thyroid supplements are NOT recommended, as they are incomplete." See more information on thyroid at www.Stopthethyroidmadness.com.

Adrenals

The adrenals produce many important hormones including DHEA, glucocorticoids such as cortisol, testosterone, and estrogen. The adrenals are highly implicated in the stress response. Low adrenal function and excess cortisol are not uncommon in autism. High cortisol can cause sleeping problems and feeling "burnt out." Excessive cortisol over time puts stress on the adrenals and can lead to adrenal fatigue. The adrenals have a relationship with the thyroid as cortisol helps get thyroid hormones from the blood to the cells for use.

Prolonged stress response may create inflammation in the brain. According to Lathe, "Stress steroids (glucocorticoids) at persistently elevated levels, first impair neuronal function in the hippocampus, and eventually cause neuronal death" (Lathe, 2006).

Symptoms of low adrenal function

The following are common symptoms that adrenal function is low:
- Fatigue
- Sleep problems, can't fall asleep, wake frequently
- Wake in morning tired
- Depression
- Cravings for carbohydrates or sugars
- Poor immune function
- Intolerance to cold

The following are symptoms of low adrenal function specific to ASD:
- Anxiety, especially with obsessive compulsive disorder (OCD)
- Poor task switching
- Sensory integration problems
- Meltdowns and tantrums
- Engaging in repetitive/stimming behaviors to escape
- Inability to tolerate people

Supporting the adrenals with adrenal glandular, B5, B6, vitamin C, and herbal formulas such as rhodiola rosea or ashwaganda is helpful. Homeopathics such as Pekana's stress kit can be helpful for supporting an exhausted and stressed system.

Pancreas

The pancreas is another important endocrine gland in autism. The pancreas regulates blood sugar and certain digestive enzymes. If the pancreas is stressed from managing blood sugar, the digestive enzymes (such as chymotrypsin an enzyme for protein digestion) may not be released sufficiently. Blood sugar regulation is essential. Bock points out that hypoglycemia is common with ASDs and discusses how insulin resistance (causing hypoglycemia) is triggered by inflammation and inflammation is high in those with ASDs (Bock, 2007). Blood sugar is often well regulated using dietary intervention of low refined carbohydrates and sugar, with increased protein and fat.

Tying it all Back to the Brain

We have learned about many problems and insufficiencies common in children with ASD. In almost all cases, these body systems which are not functioning optimally impact brain and brain function. As such, I offer a small summary relating the information offered above back to the brain.

Poor detoxification can cause the liver to produce many toxic metabolites during the process of incomplete detoxification. Poor detoxification allows for toxins, both endogenous (from within) such as produced by gut bacteria and exogenous (from without) such as mercury to accumulate. All of these toxins can affect behavior or damage brain cells.

Poor digestion can cause foods to be broken down incompletely creating opiates that affect neurotransmitters in the brain. Dysbiotic microorganisms in the gut can create toxins that affect brain function. Constipation can cause toxins to recirculate, negatively affect the brain.

Poor immune function creates inflammation, which can directly cause inflammation in the brain. An overactive Th2 response can create autoantibodies to the brain and nervous system such as autoantibodies to myelin basic protein (nerve "padding"). However, the good news is that our brains continue to myelinate until our mid-forties.

Sleep

Sleep is often a problem with children with autism. It can be due to high cortisol, and inability to manufacture or methylate melatonin, acid reflux and other digestive pain that keeps children awake.

B6 can help with sleep. Additionally, any supplements that boost methylation (B12, folinic, DMG) could be helpful if methylation was low. Make sure there is no light coming into the bedroom. Homeopathics are quite helpful for sleep.

Melatonin is often used with great success with 61% of parents stating an improvement from it (according to ARI). While I have not heard of anything negative about melatonin, there is some concern for long-term use (more than a few months). However, parents and children being sleep deprived is not good, so trying melatonin for the short term is reasonable. I suggest clients work with a physician to make any long term decision. See *Melatonin* for more thoughts on safety.

Seizures

About thirty percent of people with ASD have seizures. Patricia Murphy, former vice president of the Epilepsy Advocacy Council, states in her book that, "allopathic medicine has classified about 70 percent of cases of epilepsy as idiopathic (without any identifiable cause)." What that tells me is that there is a lot about seizures that allopathic medicine (and all of us for that matter) does not understand about seizures.

Seizures appear to have links to toxins that presumably cross into the brain. Viruses, phenols, ammonia excess, environmental toxins, and yeast toxins all seem to have an effect or are a trigger for seizures. *Of course, seizures are serious and should always involve primary care from a licensed physician.* Below you will find some information regarding diet, nutrition, and seizures. This information is not likely to be given to you by most physicians.

According to Jaquelyn McCandless, M.D., seizures have been associated with viruses including herpes simplex virus and cytomegalovirus in some people (McCandless, 2004). More research needs to be done, but I assume toxins given off by these viruses could be having a neurotoxic effect. Poor phenol processing also appears to be associated with seizures. I have one client whose seizures stopped within days of eliminating phenols (actually it was significantly reducing phenols as you can never completely remove them). According to Schauss, environmental toxins such as pesticides and industrial chemicals can be causes of seizures. Food and chemical sensitivities can play a big role—Schauss had great success with his daughter's seizures by identifying food sensitivities with a LEAP test (more about this in the *Assessments* section). Additionally, yeast overgrowth can produce a state of ammonia excess and give off neurotoxic substances. I have a client whose seizures were reduced greatly when he went on the SCD to fight yeast. In cases like this, yeast toxins appear to a contributing factor to seizures.

Additionally, low carbon dioxide ($CO2$) is also often associated with seizures. Kids presenting with suppression of $CO2$ may shun nitrogen-rich foods like meat due to the formation of ammonia (an alkaline compound of nitrogen and hydrogen) leading to a state of hyperammonemia, a highly alkaline state. In hyperammonemia, ammonia is recirculated into the blood stream instead of being discharged by the liver. It often causes brain fog, and in more serious cases, seizures. It appears to be caused by a deficiency of the amino acids citrulline, aspartic acid, threonine, and arginine. Foods rich in arginine (nuts, grains, coconut, raisins, etc.) can help reduce this ammonia. Additionally, for those who cannot break down meat, nitrogen levels can build up further. Patricia Kane suggests giving bicarbonates one hour after every meal. Some people recommend 2 ½ to 3 hours after every meal. Vitamin K Yahoo group more on bicoarbonates.

Fast breathing (either shallow or deep) is part of the stress response, which creates lack of CO2. This is another mechanism that leads to hyperammonemia. As these children are so often stressed due to hypersensitivities and physical imbalances, it would be advantageous to work with breathing and the stress response. Dr. Robert Fried has a method to work with breathing that can really help with excess ammonia production and seizures and has a book called *Breathe Well, Be Well*.

Buffered C (potassium bicarbonate, calcium carbonate, magnesium carbonate) is often supportive to these children with excess ammonia. As well, bicarbonates that are available from companies such as KTS can be helpful. However, the use of too much bicarbonate can cause the system to become overly alkaline. Alpha ketoglutarate also clears ammonia.

Butyrates also reduce the effects of abnormal nitrogen metabolism. Butyrate, (also butyric acid), found in supplement form and in butter (raw butter is particularly high), has been shown to clear ammonia and nitrogen, modulate local electrolyte flux, supports the reduction of diarrhea and improves very large, hard stools. Butyric acid also supports and fuels the intestinal walls to support a healthy gut and is used as an anticandida substance.

McCandless says taurine helps with seizures, 400-1000 mg/day and up to 2000 mg in divided doses (McCandless, 2004). Liver and gallbladder congestion are major issues in states of toxicity—taurine and butyrate ensure that your gallbladder bile flow is functional. Interestingly, Schauss explains that electrolytes are needed to transport the taurine into the brain (Schauss, 2006).

According to Owens, biotin deficiency can cause seizures (Pangborn, 2005). Assessing biotin levels through an organic acid test of B-hydroxyisovalerate and supplementing as necessary can be helpful. While some claim benefit from carnosine with seizures, Pangborn warns about some "worrisome aspects" of carnosine. See Panborn and Baker's book *Autism: Effective Biomedical Treatments* for more on carnosine.

Remember one of the most important things—look into environmental toxins around the home that may be the cause of the seizures. I had one client who moved into a home with toxic black mold and her child on the autism spectrum began having seizures after moving in.

Regarding diet, there are several diets that children have reported benefit from for seizures, apparently depending on the cause. For yeast and microbial toxins, SCD or another anti-candida diet; for artificial ingredients and phenols, Feingold Diet; for high ammonia, low protein diet; and for food sensitivity triggers, GFCF and removal of other food sensitivities. I also suspect removal of grains, lectins, and oxalates could be helpful due to their inflammatory nature. The ketogenic diet is a high fat diet created for seizure disorders. The ketogenic diet is very restrictive and must be done under the supervision of a physician, but has been helpful for some of the most severe seizures disorders. See the *ASD Diet Options* section.

Pyroluria

Pyroluria results in the abnormal production of pyrroles, which bind with B6, zinc and manganese, thus depleting these nutrients. Symptoms of pyroluria include:

- Loss of appetite.
- Motion sickness.
- Problems with sugar metabolism.
- Allergies.
- Paranoia.
- Sweet, fruity breath and body odor.
- Occasional loss of contact with reality.
- Amnesia spells.
- Low stress tolerance.

In the chapter on B6 and Zinc (and pyroluria) in his book, Nutrition and Mental Illness, Carl Pfeiffer Ph.D., M.D. discusses how zinc and B6 deficiencies are common in children with autism (Pfeiffer, 1987:45-46). Pfeiffer's and other similar work convinced Dr Bernard Rimland to look into and then study B6 supplementation with children with autism, and he found that "Behavior was rated as deteriorating significantly during the B6 withdrawal." (Rimland, 1978). William J. Walsh, Ph.D. founder and director of research of Health Research Institute and Pfeiffer Treatment Center (Warrenville, Illinois) , found 6% of a study population had a pyrrole disorder (Walsh, 2001). However, Dr. Woody McGinnis, M.D. feels that high pyrroles are found in as many as 50% of cases of ASD (Safe Harbor, 2004). Vitamin Diagnostics, a New Jersey lab, tests for urinary levels of pyrroles (see *Assessment* in *Impact of Nutrients*) and supplementation with B6 and zinc corrects the problem, often in a few weeks. It also appears pyrolurics are very often deficient in GLA, because low zinc levels make it difficult to convert LA (linoleic acid) to GLA (gamma linolenic acid). They often don't seem to need omega-3s, so this is why fatty acid testing is important. Pyroluria is discussed in more detail by Joan Mathews Larson, Ph.D in *Depression-Free Naturally* (Mathews Larson, 1999) and by Julia Ross, M.A. in *The Mood Cure*. Julia Ross, at her Recovery Systems Clinic, Mill Valley, CA has found that pyroluria prevents "full response to nutrient therapy until it is addressed," (Ross, 2002).

PART TWO

Compendium of Nutritional Strategies and Opportunity

IMPACT OF NUTRIENTS

In Part One, we looked at many of the biochemical problems encountered in ASD. Now it is time to investigate how to address those problems. I have seen in my own practice how even one or two nutrients or supplements can make a big difference in digestion, learning, or social behavior. Little by little, as nutrients are absorbed, utilized, and replenished, children often get better—progress can be slow sometimes, yet all parents welcome any improvements gladly. It is clear that by individualizing nutrition and supplementation, children can improve and even recover from autism.

This section is about understanding nutritional strategies. We will look at nutrients as supplements and within diets. We will start by talking about how nutrients supply nourishment to the body and the biochemical pathways we studied earlier. Later we will discuss each of the diets talked about in the autism community that families are using to nourish and support their children.

Common Deficiencies

Nutritional deficiencies are common in ASD. These insufficiencies lead to many of the biochemical imbalances and symptoms we see in autism. While most diets of children with autism are limited and often short on nutrients; however, even if a child were eating a nutritious and varied diet, he needs to be able to:
1. Digest the food and break it down into an absorbable form.
2. Absorb the nutrients through a healthy GI tract.
3. Convert the nutrients to usable form and utilitize them on the cellular level.

Sadly, most ASD children are unable to perform these three tasks well.

Deficiencies common in ASD include (McCandless, 2004):

- Vitamin B6
- Zinc
- Vitamin A
- Vitamins B1, B3, B5
- Biotin
- Vitamin C
- Taurine
- Selenium
- Folic acid
- Vitamin B12
- Essential fatty acid

While above I state which deficiencies are "common" in ASD, the truth is deficiencies aren't as clearcut as they have previously seemed. We see from the work of James Adams, Ph.D. that there are complexities. Adams found that levels of B6 were actually 75% higher in children with autism than control children (Adams, 2006). However, he clarifies in a 2004 study that low B6 levels are "consistent with previous studies that found that: (1) pyridoxal kinase had a very low activity in children with autism and (2) pyridoxal 5 phosphate (P5P) levels are unusually low in children with autism" (Adams 2004). In other words, while one study showed B6 was high, the level of the active form of B6, pyridoxal 5 phosphate, was low due to an inability to convert B6 to the useable form. High levels of B6 are not helpful to the body if they cannot be converted. Studies need to be looked at carefully in order to comprehend the implications of the results.

While we make generalizations about "children on the spectrum," there are always some children who have the opposite situation and fit outside the norm. While zinc deficiency is the norm, there are some rare ASD kids with copper deficiency. In these cases, giving zinc can cause problems with bleeding. We want to use the generalized information to help find trends with autism but address the needs of the individual. This is where testing and careful observation can help.

Determining Deficiencies

Half the battle is figuring out what deficiencies and imbalances are present for a child so that you can determine the best way to proceed. Laboratory testing offers a quantitative assessment of what is happening in the body. Observing symptoms as well as reactions to foods and supplements will help you get some ideas on where to start and what to test.

Functional testing, as Genova Diagnostics laboratory describes it "assesses the dynamic inter-relationship of physiological systems, thereby creating a more complete picture of one's health, unlike traditional allopathic testing, which is more concerned about the pathology of disease." Functional testing measures vitamin/mineral status, liver function of specific pathways, amino acids levels, fatty acid levels, digestive absorption, and levels of beneficial bacteria. Because of this, functional testing can help paint the picture of the individual child's health status to choose the most beneficial supplementation and dietary implementation. However, testing is definitely not perfect as it depends on human interpretation and scientific understanding (which we are expanding all of the time). Furthermore, we often have to extrapolate as testing cannot tell us everything. For example, while we can see the levels of amino acids, nutrients, and other building blocks to extrapolate the level of neurotransmitters, we cannot actually see the level of a neurotransmitter *active* in the brain.

This is where all of the detective work lies. While it can be daunting, it is one of my favorite parts of the process—seeing how all the pieces fit together. There are many "moving parts" and things don't happen in a vacuum. Piecing together the lab results with symptoms allows you to begin to undersand what to try next or what questions to ask your doctor. Over time as you understand the tests and biochemistry more, you can begin to spot good interventions to try or investigate.

You are your child's best advocate. Most importantly, you have parent's intuition, which I consider the "strongest force in the universe." Once you understand the testing and biochemistry more deeply and combine that with your knowledge of your child's day-to-day and moment-to-moment responses to things, you can begin to seek out the best supplements, diets, testing methods, and therapies.

Assessments that help determine nutritional deficiencies include: elemental/essential mineral analysis (both nutritive and toxic) through hair, urine, and/or blood, fasting amino acid analysis (plasma), and fatty acid analysis.

Assessments and Testing

The following are a list of assessments used to help uncover imbalances that might be present. Many find it helpful to look up these labs and assessments online, as it is educational to see a description of what these assessments test for and what the sample reports offer. Moreover, it becomes quite expensive to run these tests, and if you are educated you can help your physician choose the ones that might be best for your child's situation. I have listed a few labs along with the assessments to help you get started; however, it is only a partial list and I am not recommending any specific labs. It is often helpful to talk to other parents (on listservs for example) and ask them which of the tests they have found to be most helpful.

Another consideration before ordering tests is how you and your physician will alter treatments based on the results. If there are no treatments you could either begin or alter based on results, then perhaps the test will not be worthwhile, at least at the moment.

The following information for educational purposes only – it is not intended to replace medical advice. You will want to work with a physician or qualified practitioner to properly analyze and address your results.

GI Health Assessments

- **Food Sensitivity/Antibody Assessment** (blood draw or finger stick) tests IgG response for food sensitivities such as wheat, dairy, soy, corn, etc. Many companies provide this including Alletess (www.foodallergy.com), US Biotek (www.USbiotek.com), Genova Diagnostics (www.gdx.net), and Great Plains Laboratory (www.GreatPlainsLaboratory.com).
- **Inflammatory foods and substances** (blood draw) can be measured by the LEAP Test offered by Signet Diagnostic Corporation. This assessment tests for cell mediated inflammation to foods and food additives such as MSG. Instead of testing IgG response, this test assesses the actual cellular inflammatory response to foods and food additives. (www.nowleap.com).
- **Comprehensive Digestive Stool Analysis** (stool) tests digestion, absorption/assimilation, yeast overgrowth and dysbiosis. Genova Diagnostics (www.gdx.net), Doctor's Data (www.doctorsdata.com), Great Plains Laboratory (www.greatplainslaboratory.com).
- **GI Effects** (stool), GI Effects uses DNA analysis to identify microbes including anaerobic microbes, which are unavailable by culture technique. While it sounds like the best way to go to test dysbiosis, one M.D. I know who has used this test feels that the single stool sample may miss some of the microbes and makes it less effective than the classic CDSA with parasitology. Metametrix Clinical Laboratory (www.metametrix.com).
- **Intestinal Permeability** (urine) tests for leaky gut syndrome by testing for the presence of two non-metabolized sugars, lactulose and mannitol, in the urine. www.gdx.net (Genova Diagnostics), Doctor's Data (www.doctorsdata.com)
- **Celiac Disease Test** (blood) Tests for IgA human tissue transglutaminase, Serum IgA, and IgA antigliadin antibody. Genova Diagnostics (www.gdx.net), Metametrix Clinical Laboratory (www.metametrix.com). A biopsy is the definitive test for celiac but obviously more invasive.

- **Organic Acid Test** (urine) can detect byproducts of yeast, fungi, and bacteria. Tests for fatty acid metabolism, carbohydrate metabolism, cellular energy and energy production, B vitamin markers, methylation cofactor markers, neurotransmitter metabolism markers, Oxidative Damage and Antioxidant Markers, detoxification indicators. Tests for oxalates by testing oxalic acid and other organic acid markers. There is some discrepancy on the markers used to test yeast arabinose or arabinitol between the labs and yeast is notoriously difficult to test accurately. Great Plains seems to be better for oxalates and Metametrix for yeast. Great Plains Laboratory (www.greatplainslaboratory.com), Metametrix Clinical Laboratory (www.metametrix.com).
- **Beet juice test** for hydrochloric acid (home-based), this is a home-based "test" often used by Naturopathic Doctors to help determine HCl level in the stomach. Drink 1/2 cup of beet juice with a couple ounces of protein. Record the color of urine for the next six hours. The red color in beet juice is broken down by hydrochloric acid (HCl) in the stomach. If hydrochloric acid is low, urine will be a shade of light pink to red. If HCl is normal, urine is yellow in color.

Toxins and Detoxification Assessments

- **Comprehensive Detoxification Profile** (blood, saliva, and urine) assesses detoxification through for Phase I and II liver detox including sulfation. Genova Diagnostics (www.gdx.net)
- **Provocative urine test** for heavy metal toxicity (urine) tests for heavy metal toxicity including mercury. While this has been the preferred method by many doctors and DAN! practitioners, other researchers such as Andy Cutler feel that the high dose of chelator that you need to take with this test makes it dangerous. Many parents who follow the Cutler protocol prefer to test during a normal chelation round to see what the body is excreting on a regular basis. Doctor's Data (www.doctorsdata.com), Metametrix Clinical Laboratory (www.metametrix.com).
- **Hair Elements** for heavy metal toxicity (hair) tests mainly for recent heavy metal exposure and what's been excreted; however, Cutler has developed a way to interpret the minerals along with the toxic elements, giving one a good idea of toxicity (and other health issues as well) without the large chelating dose needed on provocative urine tests. Cutler's counting rules can only be applied to the hair elements test from Doctor's Data. Doctor's Data (www.doctorsdata.com), Metametrix Clinical Laboratory (www.metametrix.com).
- **Environmental Pollutants Panel** (urine) tests for levels of phthalates, benzene, styrene, and other environmental toxins in the urine. U.S. Biotek (www.usbiotek.com), Carbon Based (www.carbonbased.com) provides additional analysis of U.S. Biotek's test.
- **Porphyrins** (urine) tests for the effects of toxicity on the heme biosynthesis pathway. Based on the specific porphryins, one can get an idea of which toxins (heavy metals and environmental toxins) are present as well as whether they are having a negative effect by overburdening an organ system. Laboratoire Philippe Auguste (http://www.labbio.net/pages/index_vh_eng.htm), Metametrix Clinical Laboratory (www.metametrix.com).

Nutritional Status Assessments

- **Fatty Acid Analysis** (blood) tests the status of fatty acids (EPA, DHA, GLA, and more) along with ratios of fatty acids that are required for proper brain function, inflammatory response. Metametrix Clinical Laboratory (www.metametrix.com), Genova Diagnostics (www.gdx.net).
- **Pyroluria** (urine) tests for the binding of zinc and B6 in the body. Vitamin Diagnostics (http://www.europeanlaboratory.com/).
- **Vitamin D** (blood) tests D3, 25-Hydroxyvitamin D or 25(OH)D3, the active hormone. Metametrix Clinical Laboratory (www.metametrix.com).
- **Amino Acid Analysis** (urine or blood) tests for amino acids using urine or blood (urine is often preferred). Helps assess nutrient deficiencies, and metabolic and biochemical markers, used in methylation, to build neurotransmitter, and more uses. Metametrix Clinical Laboratory (www.metametrix.com), Genova Diagnostics (www.gdx.net), Doctor's Data (www.doctorsdata.com), Great Plains (www.greatplainslaboratory.com)
- **Minerals** (blood- erythrocyte) tests status of minerals in the blood, including intracellular which is related to nutritional status. Metametrix Clinical Laboratory (www.metametrix.com), Genova Diagnostics (www.gdx.net), Doctor's Data (www.doctorsdata.com).
- **Oxidative stress**. There are several tests for oxidative stress including CoQ10 status and lipid peroxidaton (blood-serum), and 8-hydroxy-2'-deoxyguanosine (urine), a marker of oxidative damage. Metametrix Clinical Laboratory (www.metametrix.com).
- **Vitamins** (blood) tests vitamin levels in the blood. Metametrix Clinical Laboratory (www.metametrix.com).

Hormones Assessments

- **Melatonin Analysis** (saliva) may help those with sleep disturbances by measuring melatonin, which regulates biorhythms and sleep. Genova Diagnostics (www.gdx.net),
- **Thyroid**, free T3, free T4, TSH, thyroid antibodies (blood -serum) Genova Diagnostics (www.gdx.net),
- **Adrenal** (saliva) tests cortisol and DHEA. Metametrix Clinical Laboratory (www.metametrix.com), Genova Diagnostics (www.gdx.net),

DNA Assessments

- Genovations by Genova Diagnostic lab (mouth rinse or blood) tests for methylation and other polymorphisms. www.genovations.com

Direct Laboratory Services (www.directlabs.com) is a site that does not require a doctor's prescription to get tests run. They are also available at a lower price than most doctors' offices. They carry Doctor's Data, Metametrix, and many other labs.

Your doctor or pediatrician should be willing to order the following tests to rule out genetic disorders and begin to assess biochemistry:
- Blood chemistry screen, including thyroid test (although free t3 is more reliable)
- Complete blood count (CBC)
- Urinalysis

- Serum ferritin and iron
- PKU screen (routine after birth in US hospitals)
- Chromosome studies for fragile X, Rett, Lesch-Nyhan

Getting Started with Supplements

It is common among DAN! practitioners to recommend dozens (often over 40 different) of supplements for ASD children. While you will see that many children are deficient in many nutrients and could use them in theory, sometimes too many supplements, especially if started all at once, can be problematic. If these supplements cannot be utilized—that is, if there are too many for the system to process properly— they can imbalance other nutrients or overtax the liver and kidneys. They can also imbalance the pH of the system. Additionally, if the electrolytes are out of balance, supplementation is fairly ineffective until this is corrected, as electrolytes control membrane traffic. This affects what goes in and out of the cells. While reading this paper, you may feel the need to try everything in here; however, take things slowly and seek qualified advice when necessary. More is not always better, especially with sensitive kids and an imbalanced system.

Be careful when choosing where to buy supplements. Some supplement companies can get sneaky and skimp on the actual ingredient in the product. For minerals, you want to look for elemental minerals (for example, there might be 400 mg of calcium carbonate but only 100 mg of elemental calcium). For doses of minerals below, you want the elemental level.

It is often important to take supplements in specific ways—at certain times of the day, with or without food, with or without other supplements, or in divided doses. To determine these specifics, first see what the supplement bottle recommends. If it's important to dose it a certain way, they company will often tell you. If not, I use the following rule of thumb (which is not always accurate but works in a pinch): if it's a nutrient that comes with food such as a vitamin or mineral or fatty acid, typically you take them with food. If it's an herb or an isolated amino acid, often an empty stomach is best. However, there are always exceptions. An empty stomach is about 30 minutes before a meal and 45 minutes (for a small snack) to 1½ hours after a meal (anything bigger than a snack). It is often helpful to create a schedule so you can remember when to give what. Divided doses means take the amount suggested, 100 mg for example, and divide it into doses you take two or three times a day. Water-soluble vitamins (such as vitamin C and the B-vitamins) that do not store in the system as much are best to take in divided doses. Fat-soluble vitamins (such as vitamin A and E) store in the body—so you can take them once a day if you prefer. The storage is the reason fat-soluble vitamins can cause toxicity if large amounts are taken over a period of time.

Always remember to start slowly with all supplements. Take only a small fraction (one quarter or even one tenth) of the suggested dose until you see how your child responds. Then increase it slowly over the course of four to seven days.

While I have included amounts for some of the supplements listed below, these suggestions do not address the unique needs of each child's individual biochemistry. It was a difficult decision on whether I should include these recommended amounts. Finally I decided that amounts/doses are often difficult to find so I would include them to give people a sense of a standard dose. Most are for children with ASD while others are for children in general. For specific manufacturers' products, I default to the label for optimal amounts. *This information is educational; it is not intended to treat disease.*

Vitamins

Vitamin A

Vitamin A is an antioxidant that enhances immune function; protects against infections; and affects growth, development, and protein utilization. Diarrhea—a common problem among ASD children—can be a symptom of vitamin A deficiency. According to Dr. McGinnis, PCBs cause increased breakdown of vitamin A resulting in low circulating and stored vitamin A (DAN! Syllabus, 2002:231).

Natural vitamin A, in the cis form, is important to activate T and B cells for development of long-term immune memory, for natural killer cell function, and it has a role in vision and growth of lymphoblasts (Megson, 2000). Vitamin A is crucial for proper immune function. In 1968, Scrimshaw was researching vitamin A and determined that "no nutritional deficiency in the animal kingdom is more consistently synergistic with infection than that of vitamin A" (Megson, 2000). Vitamin A deficiency increases the rate of turnover of GAGs (which aide intestinal integrity) and increases undersulfation. In a study on vitamin A levels and gut integrity, the authors state, "We found that biochemical measurements of gut integrity were best at that time of year when dietary VA [vitamin A] was most abundant. In addition, intervention with VA supplements accelerated the improvement in gut integrity in sick infants" (Thurnham, 2000).

As vitamin A is important for immune function, a chronic virus of any type may deplete stores of vitamin A. Mary Megson has used vitamin A effectively in individuals with autism that have a G-alpha protein defect when their vitamin A reserves are depleted after the DTP. Megson showed that the pertussis toxin (along with other stressors such as gluten intolerance and measles virus) can disconnect the retinoid receptors—responsible for vision, sensory perspection, language, language processing, and attention (Megson, 1999). Some studies have shown the reduction of measles when vitamin A is supplemented (Chowdhury, 2002), and another study found that chicken pox "caused an accelerated depletion of liver reserves of vitamin A" (Campos, 1987). Vitamin A is particularly helpful in vision and speech, and sideways glancing may be a sign of vitamin A deficiency and/or a G-alpha protein defect.—as it appears vitamin A may reconnect the retinoid receptors.

In one of the earliest case studies of Mary Megson's showing the efficacy of Vitamin A supplementation using cod liver oil involved a 10-year boy. A gluten-free diet and daily cod liver oil supplementation containing 5,000 IU of Vitamin A (given in divided doses of 2500 IU each) was implemented for three weeks after which a single dose of Urocholine was given. The results were remarkable. Within 30 minutes, his speech went from virtually no language to speaking a couple eight word sentences! According to Megson urocholine is "an alpha muscarinic receptor agonist, to increase bile and pancreatic secretions and indirectly stimulate hippocampal retinoid receptors." Thereafter the boy was kept on a daily dose of cod liver oil (containing 3500 IU of Vitamin A) and lower daily doses of Urocholine (12.5 mg twice a day) with continued (slow) improvement (Megson, 1999).

There are different forms of Vitamin A: the natural cis-form and the synthetic vitamin A palmitate.

Natural vitamin A is found in cod liver oil, animal liver, and animal and dairy fat from pastured animals. Megson points out from her research with autism, g-alpha protein defects, and vitamin A deficiency, "Many of these children, who need natural, unsaturated cis forms of Vitamin A found in sources such as cold water fish like salmon, or cod, liver, kidney, and milkfat, are not getting this in the modern diet. Instead, they are dependent on Vitamin A Palmitate, found in commercial infant formula and lowfat milk" (Megson, 2000). She goes on to explain that because of damage to the gut, they are not able to absorb this synthetic form. Additionally, synthetic vitamin A is not recommended, as it binds to free G-alpha protein and deactivates multiple metabolic pathways involved in vision and cell growth, disrupts hormonal regulation and metabolism of lipids, protein and glycogen (Megson, 2000).

The carotenes such as beta carotene in yellow and orange fruits and vegetables are converted in the body to vitamin A. However, some studies suggest that certain people do not do this very well (Hickenbottom, 2002). Other studies show that fat helps the conversion of beta carotene to vitamin A (Brown, 2004). For this reason, I recommend getting vitamin A directly from cod liver oil and other animal sources. I also suggest consuming carotene-rich vegetables with some good fats, such as olive oil, grapeseed oil, or any unrefined fat.

McCandless recommends 2500-5000 IU per day in a natural form (McCandless, 2004). Mary Megson recommends a vitamin A trial per Mary Megson in a conversation with Lang (Lang, 2001)) of the following:
- 2-5 years 2500 IU daily
- 5-10 years, 3750 IU daily
- 10 years plus, 5000 IU daily

Vitamin C

As we've learned from Linus Pauling, vitamin C has hundreds of uses in the body. Particularly, vitamin C plays beneficial roles with immune function. It is a powerful antioxidant along with vitamin E, selenium, and vitamin A, which neutralizes free radical damage in the gut, brain, or at the site of inflammation (common in autism). It is also helpful in reducing allergic reaction and protecting against toxins. Studies reveal that vitamin C was helpful for people with impaired glutathione synthesis (Murray, 1996:63) and people with autism often have low glutathione levels. Vitamin C was shown to raise glutathione in one study of healthy individuals by 50% (Johnston 1993). Vitamin C can be helpful to raise hydrochloric acid levels.

Since vitamin C can often be low in those with ASD, it is important to supplement. Vitamin C comes in a variety of forms. The most common is ascorbic acid, an acidic form, which can be irritating for some but helpful for those with low stomach acid. Buffered vitamin C, often sodium ascorbate or another mineral ascorbate such as magnesium ascorbate, is easier on the stomach.

Vitamin C is often made from corn so corn sensitive people should be aware of this. Also, be aware that vitamin C supplementaton can make oxalic acid appear high on laboratory testing, causing you to believe oxalates are a problem, when they may not be.

For children, 1000 mg or more. Vitamin C has low toxicity and can be taken up to bowel tolerance— which means increasing the dose by 250-500 mg per day until diarrhea occurs. Be sure to give Vitamin C in divided doses as it is water-soluble and does not remain in the body for long. After reaching bowel tolerance, decrease the dose slightly to obtain the maximum dose for that individual. It is good to note that many parents use high doses of Vitamin C when constipation is a problem, because of the effect it can have on the bowels.

Vitamin E

Vitamin E is a fat-soluble antioxidant that prevents free radical damage. It protects the lipid portion of the cell membrane from mercury and other heavy metals and toxins, protects the thymus gland and white blood cells from damage, protects the immune system from damage during chronic viral infections, protects the liver from damage, and protects polyunsaturated fats like flax and fish oil from oxidative damage (for this reason it is important that parents giving their children flax or fish oil also provide vitamin E supplementation). Vitamin E helps spare glutathione.

Look for a natural vitamin E (read the label to ensure it says "d" form, not "dl") with mixed tocopherols, including gamma tocopherol and alpha tocopherol. Vitamin E is often made from soy; however, Kirkman and New Beginnings make a soy-free form. The recommended dosage ranges from 100-400 IU (Bock, 2007) and 200-600 IU per day (McCandless, 2004).

Vitamin B6

The relationship between vitamin B6 (in combination with magnesium) and brain disorders has been studied extensively, as well as how B6 supplementation can improve neurological conditions.. Bernard Rimland, Ph.D., the pioneer in biomedical treatment for autism, lead extensive research into B6 for autism. In one of his early studies, Rimland gave 150 children with autism "megadoses" of B6 (between 150-450 mg) and saw 45% of the children had a "definite improvement."

In a double blind, crossover study published in *Biological Psychiatry*, Vitamin B6 was found to be more effective than methylphenidate (Ritalin) in a group of hyperactive children (Zimmerman, 1999:153). Tapan Audhya, Ph.D., observed that greater than 40% of autistic children had low B6, but after supplementation that number decreased to around 5% (DAN! Syllabus, 2002:241). In one study, Dr. Audhya demonstrated a ten-fold increased need for B6 among those with autism (DAN! Syllabus, 2002). James Adams, Ph.D., in his pilot study on multivitamin/mineral supplement in 2004 stated, "The finding of high vitamin B(6) levels is consistent with recent reports of low levels of pyridoxal-5-phosphate and low activity of pyridoxal kinase (i.e., pyridoxal is only poorly converted to pyridoxal-5-phosphate, the enzymatically active form). This may explain the functional need for high-dose vitamin B(6) supplementation in many children and adults with autism" (Adams, 2004). This pilot study is backed up by a similar 2006 study (Adams, 2006).

For most children on the spectrum, their ability to convert B6 to pyridoxal-5-phosphate (P5P), the active (phosphorylated) form of Vitamin B6, is reduced. However, P5P often is not tolerated in those with sulfation challenges. Additionally, be sure to take B6 with magnesium.

The dose for B6 can vary widely, Bock suggests 100 to 500 mg of B6 with 20 percent as P5P (Bock, 2007). McCandless recommends much smaller amounts, 50 mg under 5 years old and 50-100 mg per day for children over 5 years of age (McCandless, 2004).

B6 and Magnesium

Magnesium should be given with B6. Several studies by Bernard Rimland Ph.D. (author of *Infantile Autism*, the first book that recognized autism as a biological disorder as opposed to being due to "cold mothering") have shown that, used in combination, B6 and magnesium can be very effective in ASD. In 1964, Rimland began conducting studies on vitamin therapy for children with ASD. In one study, 30-40% of children showed significant improvement with few side effects when B6 was given (Shaw, 1998:177). The side effects, of irritability, sound sensitivity, and bed-wetting, cleared up when magnesium was added. In fact, the magnesium brought about improved speech and behavior (Shaw, 1998:178). In one large study by Rimland, 43% of parents reported that vitamin B6 and magnesium had been helpful, benefiting 136 out of 318 children (Rimland, 1988:S69). See more under *Magnesium*.

Vitamin B12

Vitamin B12 is required for cell formation, energy metabolism, immune function, nerve function, proper digestion, protein synthesis, and metabolism of carbohydrates and fats. Methyl B12, or methylcobalamin, is a methyl donor, as the name implies. According to Sidney Baker, M.D., a pediatrician specializing in autism and complex chronic conditions, it should be administered through an injection in order to be most effective (Pangborn and Baker, 2002:207). According to McCandless, if the effect is positive it should be noticed within a few days (McCandless, 2004). Dr. Neubrander is a doctor highly experienced in MB12 shots. See his site, www.drneubrander.com for information and stories. ARI's parent survey states that parents reported improvement with methyl-B12 63% of the time. I often hear from parents that the methyl B12 shots offered the greatest benefit to their child. However, there is a group that it's not helpful for. Yasko's approach is to use hydroxocobalamin for a group of people who don't do well with methylcobalamin.

MB12 comes in the form of sublingual tablets and if it is preferred by the parent, McCandless says "high oral doses" can be tried, although she caveats it with, "after a while [on injections]" (McCandless, 2004). Lang suggests 800 mcg per day. According to a mom I know using Dr. Patricia Kane's protocol, Kane recommends 1000 mcg B12 sublingually five times a day. That sounds like a lot to me, but I think the concept of sublingual B12 given several times throughout the day seems like a good recommendation, even if you do less.

Folic acid

Folic acid, or folate, is essential for DNA synthesis and red blood cell formation. Folic acid is often low in those with ASD (McCandless, 2002:118), and diarrhea (common in individuals with autism) can cause folate deficiency. Folic acid is best combined with B12. Folic acid is a methyl donor that helps recycle methionine for proper methylation.

Folic acid needs to be converted to 5-methyl tetrahydrofolate (5-MTHF) in the body. Many children do not have the necessary nutrients and adequate biochemical processing to make the necessary conversions. As such, many children take folinic acid–which is further along the pathway making it easier for it to get into the proper form and be utilitized. Even further along the pathway and better tolerated still is FolaPro by Metagenics which is in the most active and usable form, L-5-MTHF.

McCandless recommends 600-1000 mg of folic acid per day (McCandless, 2004) and Bock 800-1600 mg per day in whatever form is best tolerated (Bock, 2007). The higher range can be helpful if B12 is overstimulating.

Inositol

A deficiency in central nervous system (CNS) availability of inositol may produce altered brain signaling and eventually lead to the development of neurological disorders. Inositol is effective in helping to treat depression and panic disorders, since it is required for the function of serotonin and other neurotransmitters.

Inositol also appears to be very helpful for Obsessive Compulsive Disorder (OCD). William Walsh, senior research scientist, Pfeiffer Treatment Center, states, "Inositol is usually very helpful for undermethylated, high histamine. This includes nearly every OCD patient we have seen. Inositol usually provides calming throughout the day and ability to settle down to sleep at night, for these patients." (AlternativeMentalHealth.com)

IP-6, inositol hexaphosphate, is helpful for the immune system by increasing natural killer (NK) cell function. It protects the body against toxins and attaches to heavy metals such as mercury, lead and cadmium. [Ou, 1999]

I have heard from one parent that inositol alone did wonders for her child.

Biotin

Biotin is a B vitamin produced by good bacteria. If beneficial bacteria in the gut is low (as is the case for many with ASD), this nutrient may be in short supply, as beneficial flora produces biotin. Hence, children with a history of antibiotics may be low in biotin. Biotin is one of the necessary nutrients needed for the delta-6 desaturase enzyme needed to convert fatty acids to usable forms, for example converting ALA to EPA and DHA. Biotin can also be helpful for fighting yeast as it appears to be able to inhibit the conversion of benign yeast into more invasive fungal forms. Biotin deficiency can cause seizures.

74

It can be helpful to take biotin with inositol so it's easier on the liver.

Vitamin D

Vitamin D is a prohormone, a precursor to a hormone. New research shows that vitamin D does much more than we previously thought including cutting the risk of cancer significantly. In studies, researchers found vitamin D had a positive effect on reducing cancer (Garland, 2006) including one study that stated, "Providing 1,000 IU of vitamin D per day for all adult Americans would cost about $1 billion; the expected benefits for cancer would be in the range of $16-25 billion in addition to other health benefits of vitamin D." (Grant, 2007) Vitamin D increases immune activity and regulates (suppresses) it to prevent autoimmune reactions. It keeps bones strong, aids mineral absorption, and supports a healthy nervous system.

Another study, in addition to showing a decrease in deadly cancers, showed a decrease in the rates of autoimmune disorders such as rheumatoid arthritis and type 1 diabetes with vitamin D. (Holick, 2004). Vitamin D also supports the immune system and helps reduce inflammation by "suppressing inflammatory T cell activity" (Deluca, 2001). The vitamin D hormone stimulates transforming growth factor TGFbeta-1 and interleukin 4 (IL-4) production, which in turn may suppress inflammatory T cell activity

Vitamin D is manufactured by humans from sunlight in contact with the skin. Holick, from the study above on autoimmune disorders, mentions how moderate sun exposure is valuable in contributing to total vitamin D levels, stating, "Sensible sun exposure (usually 5-10 min of exposure of the arms and legs or the hands, arms, and face, 2 or 3 times per week) and increased dietary and supplemental vitamin D intakes are reasonable approaches to guarantee vitamin D sufficiency." However, Sally Fallon and the Weston A. Price organization feel that because of the northern latitude that many of us in American and Europe are on, we do not have enough direct hours of sunlight to make adequate leveles of vitamin D from the sun.

Vitamin D can also be obtained through animal fat (only from animals raised on pasture with access to sunlight) such as butter and dairy, fat from beef and lamb, and lard. Cod liver oil also contains vitamin D. However, in cod liver oil depending on the brand, the level is often pretty low–one tenth as much compared to vitamin A.

Exposure to 20 minutes of sun on exposed skin is helpful in creating some vitamin D; however, there's controversy on how much. and may require supplementation.

Depending on the diet, vitamin D supplementation may be necessary. Julia Ross recommends (for adults) testing for vitamin D (see *Assessments* in *Impact of Nutrients*) before supplementing with more than 400 IU (Ross, 2002). With that said, the earlier study showed the increased benefit to the population with 1000 IU—more needs to be learned about optimum levels. This is an area with a lot of new study currently, and I'd suspect more information may be coming out soon with revised vitamin D supplementation levels for children and adults. Be sure to add total amount of vitamin D from other supplements such as cod liver oil. Bio-D-Mulsion by Biotics Research is an absorbable form of emulsified oil that contains 400 IU vitamin D in one drop, and Bio-D-Mulsion Forte with 2000 IU in one drop.

Vitamin K

Vitamin K is a fat-soluble vitamin. Vitamin K is known to be important in blood coagulation (clotting) and bone metabolism. Today we are discovering many more uses for vitamin K as well as the interplay between vitamin K and vitamins A and D. Vitamin K is a powerful antioxidant, inhibits inflammatory cytokines, and aids in the development of the nervous system.

Vitamin K1 is found in leafy greens, broccoli, lettuce, cabbage, spinach and green tea. It's also found in olive oil and hemp oil (many foods high in oxalates). Vitamin K2 is found in pastured animal fats such as egg yolk, butter, liver, certain cheeses; fermented soybean products such as natto; and appears to be the most active form for the effects on calcium and bone metabolism (Zitterman). Vitamin K is produced by beneficial bacteria; as such it would make sense that children on the spectrum, many with dysbiosis, would not have enough vitamin K.

There is a group of parents and researchers studying vitamin K for its effects on regulating glutamate toxicity in the brain and the theory that deficiency is the cause of the calcium oxalate crystals found in many autistic children. Vitamin K is important to the development of bone proteins that control calcium and may influence cellular firing and glutamate toxicity as well as tight gut junctions. Vitamin K may help control the liver's production of oxalic acid, so that low vitamin K may cause the body to increase its own production of oxalic acid. Oxalate-rich foods are also high in vitamin K, and as we reduce oxalates, we reduce vitamin K from these plant sources such as leafy greens. Also, if beneficial bacteria that normally produce vitamin K is low, this would make vitamin K levels even lower. Vitamin K appears to chelate calcium from the crystals and be an important piece of the puzzle. See the yahoo group http://health.groups.yahoo.com/group/VitaminK/ for extensive discussion and files regarding the use of Vitamin K in ASD.

Multivitamin/mineral formula

When a wide range of vitamins and minerals are well tolerated, a multivitamin/mineral formula can be a good supplement to use as. They contain a wide variety of nutrients—helpful as people with ASD often have multiple deficiencies. Multivitamin/mineral formulas can be good for children who are averse to taking a lot of supplements as there is only one supplement. However, on the downside, multivitamins often have a strong flavor due to the B-vitamins, also making it difficult to give them to smell-sensitive and picky eaters. Multis can also make it difficult to determine exactly which nutrients are helping and which may be creating a negative reaction. Dr. Kenneth Bock in his book, *Healing the New Childhood Epidemics: Autism ADHD, Asthma and Allergies*, recommends only giving multis if the child has already demonstrated an ability to tolerate a number of supplements without any negative reactions (Bock, 2007).

There are dozens of companies that make multivitamin/mineral formulas for children; however, most of them (especially the good tasting ones) are loaded with sugar, artificial colors, and other additives that many ASD children should avoid. Look for a company that formulates its product specificially for autistic spectrum disorders. They often use better absorbable and usable forms of nutrients, in combinations that are needed children with ASD. For example, many do not add copper (as zinc is in short supply in the body), use non-constipating forms of iron, use folinic instead of folic acid, and add other specialty nutrients such as DMG. Additionally, many products formulated for autism make sure to avoid artificial ingredients and salicylates.

BrainChild Nutritionals, formulated by Michael Lang, researcher and father of two autistic children, contain no salicylates or phenols (for those with faulty sulfation), no sugars, colors, artificial ingredients of any kind. In addition to highly absorbable nutrients, they contain herbs to soothe and heal the gut, aid in detoxification, and support proper organ function. Moreover, the most unique aspect about them is that they contain many different sources of easy to absorb, non-reactive sulfates including MSM, biotin, thiamine, and NAC. If you suspect cysteine and/or other forms of sulfate are not processing properly, look for symptoms of a toxic build up including violence, rash, anxiety, wheezing, nausea, cramps, and diarrhea. New Beginnings, Kirkman, and Learner's Edge are also companies that make multivitamin/mineral formulations specificially for autistic spectrum disorders.

Minerals

Magnesium

Magnesium deficiency in children is characterized by excessive fidgeting, anxious restlessness, psychomotor instability, and learning difficulties in the presence of normal IQ, according to Seelig (Block, 2002). Magnesium is helpful for energy production and in enzyme activation. Magnesium is used in over 300 enzyme systems and is a very important mineral. Magnesium aids with muscle relaxation, sleep, tics, and anxiety and depression. Magnesium can also help with constipation. Magnesium in the forms of magnesium citrate and magnesium sulfate are great for constipation, and magnesium oxide firms up stools. According to Rimland, magnesium glycinate and magnesium citrate are the most absorbable forms.

Magnesium can also be absorbed through the skin through Epsom salt (magnesium salt) baths, discussed further in Appendix VII on phenols. Make sure to account for Epsom salt baths when supplementing with magnesium. While I'd assume you cannot get a toxic dose transdermally, the combination of transdermal and oral may be too much for your child—the most obvious sign of that is diarrhea. . For children who tend to drink the bath water, they may get diarrhea from the Epsom salt.

Magnesium at 200-350 mg per day in divided doses is a common recommendation and Dr. Rimland (one of the pioneers with B6 and magnesium) suggested 4mg of magnesium per pound of body weight (eg. 400 mg for 100 pound person).

Zinc

A zinc deficiency may make children irritable, tearful, sullen and have gaze aversion, according to Moynahan (Block, 2002). Deficiency can cause susceptibility to infection and inflammation, decrease in T cell count, growth retardation, inflammatory bowel disease, and loss of appetite (Murray, 1996:184-5). White lines in fingernails, retarded growth, poor taste and smell, excema, and poor wound healing are signs of zinc deficiency. Zinc deficiency can result from protein deficiency, diarrhea, and chelation of heavy metals (Murray, 1996:184-5), which are fairly common circumstances in autistic children. According to Tapan Audhya, a Ph.D. focused on Neuro-Endocrinology and Nutritional Biochemistry, over 40% of autistic children had low zinc compared with controls. Additionally, William Walsh Ph.D., studied 503 children with autism and discovered that 85% had high copper-zinc ratios. Because zinc competes with copper for absorption, this high ratio is a sign that zinc is deficient and copper is in excess (McCandless, 2002:124).

Zinc supplementation can improve immune system function, enzymatic processes, sensory function, appetite, and cell growth.

The body can bind zinc and B6 in a condition called pyroluria (as discussed in more detail above). If a child has this condition, zinc and B6 cannot be utilized properly and higher doses would be necessary to compensate. You can have your child tested for this condition (see Assessments in Impact of Nutrients section).

It's rare, but a few ASD kids are copper deficient. They will get nosebleeds from dosing zinc. I must emphasize it is rare, but it happens, so as with every supplement go slowly and be observant.

Give zinc between meals or at bedtime so it is not taken with other nutrients such as calcium, folic acid, and iron that can inhibit absorption. Also take zinc away from phosphorylated nutrients such as P5P. Zinc inactivates DPP-IV, so take it two hours away from food and enzymes that contain DPP-IV. Because of this, Pangborn cautions against giving the full days dose with one meal. Be aware that zinc (typically zinc sulfate) can cause nausea on an empty stomach.

For some children who have a difficult time taking zinc, zinc picolinate seems to be more bioavailable and a form with less side effects for some children, and according to William Walsh of the Pfeiffer Treatment Center, zinc picolinate is good for poor GI tracts; however, it can be a problem for children with excitotoxic sensitivity . Zinc methionine is another form that seems to have superior absorption. Zinc sulfate is a bioavailable form, although can cause stomach upset. Zinc citrate and zinc acetate are also good forms.

According to Pangborn, the "low dose level" starts at 5 mg. Amount range based on age. While the FDA DRI (dietary reference intake) is 15 mg/day, many children on the autism spectrum, appear to need more. A common dose of zinc for children with ASD is 25-50 mg; however, some children seem to need a lot more especially those with high copper levels or for some bigger kids. McCandless recommends one milligram per pound of body weight. Divided doses seem to work best for most children.

78

Calcium

As many people know, calcium is important for bones and teeth, as it is a major component of bone synthesis. It is also important for muscle contraction, blood pressure, blood coagulation, energy production, immune system function, and nerve conduction.

However, most do not realize how important calcium is for brain function. Calcium regulates the speed, intensity, and clarity of every message that passes between neurons. Calcium signals the uptake and release of neurotransmitters. Calcium also interacts with potassium and sodium to maintain proper levels of nerve-cell stimulation, which balances nerve cell activation and inactivation in the brain. Calcium also interacts with zinc in the regulation of histamine (a neurotransmitter) and is dependent on DHA (a fatty acid that is commonly low in autistic children) for all membrane functions.

Lead competes for calcium binding sites, according to Dr. Woody McGinnis, MD (DAN! Syllabus, 2002:234). Additionally, the Standard American Diet (SAD), full of sugar, soda, and processed foods, is highly acidic and leaches calcium from the body's supply (bones and tissue) to neutralize the acid.

Since many children with autism have dairy sensitivities, it is important to supplement with calcium and attempt to consume **non-dairy sources** such as: leafy greens, almonds (almond milk and almond butter), sunflower seeds, sesame seeds (sesame butter/tahini), beans, blackstrap molasses, lamb, carob, figs, and broccoli. Because kids are not thrilled with many of these foods, try chopping the greens in a food processor and hiding them in tomato sauce, or add seaweed whole to cooking rice or soup and remove it before eating.

Successful calcium supplementation is a little complex, as it requires magnesium, vitamin D, and vitamin K for optimal absorption. Supplemental calcium in the form of calcium carbonate is not very absorbable, and calcium citrate or calcium bound to other Kreb cycle intermediates (such as calcium malate) are preferred (Murray, 1996); however, some children may have trouble with the aspartate form as it can have neurotoxic effects similar to glutamate.

According to McCandless, children need from 800-1200 mg of calcium daily from a combination of food and supplement sources (McCandless, 2002).

Selenium

Selenium is a trace mineral and antioxidant that, with vitamin E, helps prevent free radical damage. It is important for immune function, as it is used in glutathione peroxidase in the formation of white blood cells and increases the activity of natural killer cells. According to Dr. Haley, selenium neutralizes mercury (DAN! 2002) and is a helpful nutrient for mercury detoxification and important during chelation. In a study at Istanbul's Medical University, selenium was shown to protect neuron message transmission due to the prevention of free radical damage (Zimmerman, 1999:151). According to Dr. Audhya, over 60% of autistic children have low RBC (red blood cell) selenium (DAN!, 2002).

Selenium can be toxic in excess, so dosing should be a total of 100-200 mcg/day (McCandless, 2002:125). Be sure to use the selenomethionine form. If you are avoiding yeast, be sure to verify that you use a yeast-free brand.

Amino Acids

DMG (Dimethylglycine) and TMG (Trimethylglycine)

DMG is a methyl donor, as is TMG, also called betaine after it was identified in beets. TMG has two methyl donors and after it donates a methyl group becomes DMG. As we saw in methylation, TMG can donate a methyl group (instead of folic acid) to recycle homeocysteine to methionine.

The Autism Research Institute has been gathering data for 20 years on autistic children who have tried DMG. There has been no evidence of toxic effect nor any significant adverse effects from DMG (Shaw, 1998:193). Additionally, the *Journal of Laboratory and Clinical Medicine* states that DMG is a "natural, simple compound with no known undesirable side effects" (Shaw, 2998:188). In laboratory rabbits, DMG increased immune system function by 300-1000%. Although no clinical trials have been done on DMG for improving speech in autistic children, many parents and clinicians have seen great results. Lee Dae Kun, Director of the Pusan (Korea) Research Center on Child Problems tried the supplement on 39 children with ASD of which 80% had positive results, such as improved speech, eating, excretion, and willingness (Shaw, 1998:192).

If DMG substance is going to work for an individual, its results are usually seen within a week. According to McCandless, 50% of children who take DMG benefit. She suggests starting with one 125 mg sublingual tablet of DMG, and working up to six (McCandless, 2004). TMG, trimethylglycine, at 500-800 mg/ day is an option if DMG doesn't work; however, some parents noticed hyperactivity with TMG (McCandless, 2004). Shaw suggests starting with a 3-4 week trial—starting with 1/2 of a 125 mg tablet for a pre-school aged child and one 125 mg tablet for a larger child. Increase the dose to 1-4 tablets per day for children and 2 to 8 for adults (Shaw, 1998). In *Autism: Effective Biomedical Treatments* by Pangborn and Baker, there is a detailed chart on how to choose DMG or TMG and well as whether to add B12 and folic acid.

NAC (N-acetyl cysteine)

N-acetyl cysteine, a sulfur-bearing conjugated amino acid, is converted in the body to cysteine and glutathione.

NAC is a way to supplement glutathione, as it is converted to glutathione and the body can utilize it more readily. Glutathione is depleted in autistic children, as it is used up to combat many free radical and damaging processes. According to Dr. Audhya, Ph.D., almost 46% of autistic children have levels of glutathione that are below normal (DAN! Syllabus, 2002, 240).

NAC can be used to neutralize toxins (Lang, 2000:4). Free radicals generated by yeast toxins (gliotoxins) can be neutralized by NAC or glutathione, along with vitamin C, vitamin E, and lipoic acid (Shaw,

1998:105). Hospitals use NAC to neutralize an acetaminophen (phenol) overdose, and it has been used successfully by Lang to counter phenol exposure ("overdose") in those who are sensitive. Additionally, from research by Breitkreutz and Hack, NAC helped AIDS patients to regain NK activity and combat T cell cytotoxicity (Breitkreutz 2000)—both immune problems seen in autism.

Lang suggests small doses of 20-40 mg daily if faulty sulfation is suspected (Lang, 2002).

Glutathione

Glutathione is an essential substance. Glutathione is a powerful antioxidant and detoxifying agent. Glutathione aids the immune system and repairs the gut. However, glutathione is not absorbed and utilized effectively by the body when it is supplemented orally. Liposomal glutathione (basically glutathione wrapped in a fat molecule), appears to be more effective. IV glutathione is much more utilized by the body, and available only through physicians.

Amino Acid Formulas

Amino acids are the building blocks for proteins and are important in muscle and tissue growth and repair, neurotransmitters, immune responses, enzymes, and detoxification. Some amino acids we can synthesize, others must be consumed through food and are called essential amino acids. Amino acids can be very powerful and an important piece of the puzzle.

Methionine, cysteine and glutathione are needed for the methylation and transsulfuration pathways. Glutamine, for example, can help heal the gut lining, build/repair muscle, and function as "brain fuel" when glucose is not available.

Taurine aids digestion of fat, as it is used to produce bile salts for digestion of fat. When taurine is in short supply, seizures can result. Taurine has been shown to help decrease blood sugar in diabetics.

Carnitine aids fatty acid metabolism, sending the fat to the mitochondria of the cell to be burned. This allows for fats to be utilitized better, increasing energy production (reducing fatigue), decreasing triglycerides and cholesterol in the blood, and reducing fatty acid oxidation.

Glycine is an amino acid that is very helpful in detoxifying industrial chemicals.

These are just a few of the important amino acids and help to illustrate the importance and benefit of supplementing them properly.

Essential amino acids need to be taken in, from the diet or supplementation. Non-essential amino acids are created by the body if it is functioning properly and has the right building blocks; however, that may not be the case in autism.

An amino acid analysis (for testing information see Assessments in Impact of Nutrients section) is an important step to determining which amino acids are low for the individual child, and what nutrients and coenzymes are deficient or adequate. Supplementation should be done accordingly, cautiously, and slowly.

Custom blends are often a good way to go, and various labs identify and offer custom formulations based on individual needs. These are often helpful and more successful than the kind of amino acid blends you can purchase at the health food store.

Protein and amino acids are complicated with ASD. Many children with ASD are not consuming enough protein and/or don't have the right enzymes to break down the protein properly. Additionally, amino acids need metabolic (not digestive) enzymes to convert from one form to another to be utilitized by the body, as we saw with the methionine cascade. For enzymes to convert the amino acids, many nutrients are often needed especially magnesium, necessary in over 300 different enzymes. With low nutrient reserves in the ASD population, this conversion often does not happen. Supplementation can cause a build up of an intermediate metabolite, most frequently resulting in regressive symptoms. While custom blends individualize amino acid supplementation (which is beneficial), they do not fix the problem of potential intermediate metablites forming in children that may have an inability to properly convert them.

Another challenge with amino acid supplementation is that amino acids compete for absorption. Supplementing them, especially with single amino acids, can throw off the essential balance (Lang, 2002).

According to McCandless, two-thirds of children with ASD have an abnormal amino acid profiles. Taurine, cysteine, and glutamine are the three that tend to be low (McCandless, 2004): however, proceed with caution as cysteine and glutamine are excitotoxins (substances that can excite brain cells, even leading to cell death). Glutamine and glutamate are neuroexcitatory amino acids and can cause hyperactivity and excitatory behavior is some children. This sort of negative response can be fairly prolonged, even after stopping the supplements. Amy Yasko, N.D., Ph.D. specializing in autistic spectrum disorders, warns strongly against neuroexcitatory amino acids as they can excite neurons to death in some people. She cautions against the use of glutamate, glutamine, aspartate, and to a lesser extent cysteine and homocysteine. Glutamate converts into GABA, and these two neurotransmitters regulate the opening (glutamate) and closing (GABA) of the calcium channel allowing the cell to fire. Vitamin B6 is an important coenzyme in the conversion of glutamate to GABA. A B6 deficiency may be one reason why children with autism have glutamate excess. There also may be a relationship with vitamin K in preventing neuroexcitotoxicity. Additionally, metallothinoneins (poorly functioning in autism) can protect brain cells from glutamate-induced toxicity. Definitely avoid dietary sources of monosodium glutamate (MSG). However, as a generalization, whether to take or not take glutamate or glutamine, is a difficult question to answer, as amino acid supplementation is often very helpful for kids with ASD.

As with any supplement, one should watch for any changes in behavior. Please note, that if supplementation is stopped because of an adverse reaction, it may still take several days for the behavior to settle, as these amino acids stay in the body and affect processes for quite a while. If this happens,

82

check with your health care provider—typically you will want to build up nutrient reserves that will help convert the amino acids for several months before trying amino acids again.

Essential Fatty Acids

Omega-3

Omega-3 is found in fish oil, cod liver oil (also high in vitamin A and D), and flax seeds/oil. There are few good sources of omega-3 in the Standard American Diet or food supply (unless you are able to get pastured animal products), which translates into low concentrations in breast milk (Stoll, 2001:101). Omega-3 is crucial for cognitive function and brain development. Omega-3 also helps reduce inflammation—often present in the gut of autistic children. Additionally, Dr. Stoll cites many studies showing fish oil's positive benefits in alleviating attention deficit (Stoll, 2001:157). Omega-3 can also help boost Th1 lymphocytes, allowing the immune system to defend against viruses and other infections.

In the body, the essential fatty acid ALA (alpha-linolenic acid) found in flax seed is converted to EPA with the enzyme delta 6 desaturase, after which it is converted to DHA. Because of a variety of reasons (excess insulin, poor digestion, etc.) some people are not able to efficiently convert ALA to EPA and ultimately DHA. Because those with autism often have many health challenges and poor digestion, I recommend fish oil over flax oil. Additionally, flax oil was shown to increase the risk of prostate cancer in one study (Lietzmann, 2004). Dr. Stoll points out all of the studies on omega-3's effects on psychiatric illnesses have involved fish oil, not flax. It is important to research which companies have good quality controls for fish oil (like Nordic Naturals, Coromega), as it can contain mercury naturally occurring in fish.

Cod liver oil differs from fish oil, in that cod liver oil (as the name implies) is from the liver of the codfish making it high in vitamin A and D, fish oil is from the fish body and does not contain vitamins A and D. Additionally, the ratio of fatty acids is different. Cod liver oil is higher in DHA and fish oil is higher in EPA. To generalize, DHA is particularly good for the brain including the function of brain cell receptors, which allow the entry of important neurological chemicals including neurotransmitters and hormones. EPA is very good for reducing inflammation and often used in depression.

In order to utilize and balance omega-3 and omega-6, it is essential that you eliminate all trans fats. Trans fats fit in the essential fatty acid receptor sites and imbalance/compete with the good fats. Trans fats are found in commercial margarine, commercial peanut butter, and any hydrogenated oil.

Dr. McCandless recommends 500-1000mg EPA and 250-500 mg of DHA per day (McCandless, 2004). According to James Adams in the *Summary of Biomedical Treatments for Autism*, he recommends 20-60 mg/kg of omega-3 (600-1800 mg for a 60 lb child). Adams further suggests a supplement richer in DHA for younger children, and a supplement richer in EPA for older children and adults. Cod liver oil is naturally higher in DHA and fish body oils are higher in EPA. Make sure to distinguish between milligrams of omega-3 (EPA and DHA) verses milligrams of "fish oil." 1000 mg of fish oil, may only have 550 mg of omega-3. Typically recommendations are given based on milligrams of omega-3 (EPA or DHA) although the front of the label may measure it in milligrams of fish oil.

Omega-6 and GLA

While omega-3 is recommended for everyone, omega-6 may or may not be as beneficial depending on the individual, because the Standard American Diet provides far too much omega-6 (typically linoleic acid or LA) compared to omega-3. It is important to consider, however, if your child has been eating the Standard American Diet. All omega-6 fatty acids are not equal. Most vegetable oils (such as canola, corn and others generally found in processed foods) are high in the omega-6 fatty acid LA but very low in GLA. Gamma linolenic acid (GLA) is an omega-6 fatty acid that converts to PGE1 (a prostaglandin) and is anti-inflammatory in nature. It can have powerful effects on brain function and reduction of inflammation. The body can convert LA into GLA however it requires the same delta-6 desaturase enzyme (and all of the other factors) for conversion as converting the omega-3s's from ALA to DHA and EPA. We often have too much LA and not enough GLA. The main sources of GLA are evening primrose oil, borage oil, and black currant seed oil, hemp seed oil, and spirulina. The only substantial food based GLA I have found are hemp seeds and hemp seed oil. In fact, hemp seeds are much higher in complete protein than other nuts and seeds (right up there with soybeans and twice that of almonds), have the ideal ratio of omega-6 to omega-3 (4:1), and are a wonderful source of GLA. You can find hemp seeds and hemp oil in the vitamin department of any natural food store. They are good tasting and great to eat plain or sprinkle on crackers with almond butter. Do not confuse hemp seeds with hemp flour, as they do not share the same nutritional benefits. Hemp seeds contain the beneficial oil and protein, while the flour is often made from the husks containing little nutrition.

Bock recommends 80-240 mg GLA (Bock, 2006). McCandless' recommendation of GLA is 50-100 mg (McCandless, 2004).

Make sure you consume enough vitamin E so the fats do not oxidize in the body (see vitamin E in the vitamin section).

Omega-9

This is an important fatty acid, but not actually an "essential" fatty acid as our bodies can manufacture it so it's not "essential" to get it from food. With that said, omega-9 is an important fatty acid and getting some in the diet is healthy. Omega-9 has heart protective benefits, helps prevent oxidation of cholesterol, and may be beneficial with cancer. Omega-9 supplementation is usually not necessary given the high amount of it in the diet and our ability to manufacture it.

Fatty Acid Balance

Doing a fatty acid panel is very helpful to determine fatty acid status of omega-3s, 6s and other fats. Supplementing is more accurate and successful after you know where your child is. Many of the omega-3 and omega-6 oils require an enzyme (metabolic not digestive) called delta 6 desaturase. Depending on the EFA, high levels on test results may indicate (1) too much of the fatty acid in the diet, or (2) not enough of this enzyme to break it down and the EFA pathway gets "stuck." Delta 6 desaturase can be blocked by too many polyunsaturated oils, thyroid insufficiency, high blood sugar or insulin, or viruses.

84

Additionally, this enzyme needs enough vitamin A, E, B6, B12, niacin, biotin, magnesium, zinc, selenium, manganese, and sulfur. See Assessments earlier in this section for which tests to help with determining these levels.

GI Supplements

Digestive Enzymes

Digestive enzymes are one of the most beneficial supplements and one of the first things I recommend for clients, unless the child has serious gut inflammation or an ulcer. Firstly, enzymes help break down food for better digestion. Using enzymes can reduce gas, bloating, constipation, and diarrhea. A high quality enzyme product with good proteases will break down the proteins to reduce and prevent reactions to foods. Enzymes can also help avoid the development of new food sensitivities by breaking down proteins that create an inflammatory response or other negative reaction. Enzymes help reduce hyperactivity caused by food sensitivities (Lee, 1998:116). Furthermore, enzymes break down foods properly so they don't feed the yeast and bad bacteria, thereby reducing inflammation and leaky gut. Enzymes such as protease and cellulose taken on an empty stomach can also break down the cell wall of yeast and viruses to kill them and make them vulnerable to other yeast killing agents or the immune system.

When taken on an empty stomach, enzymes can help reduce circulating inflammatory proteins in the bloodstream, as well as breakdown yeast and viruses. When there is inflammation anywhere in the body (gut inflammation, headache, tendonitis), it is created by inflammatory proteins—or prostaglandins. Enzymes, especially proteases or proteolitic enzymes on an empty stomach, will break down these inflammatory proteins floating around in the blood stream.

The most simple and common use of enzymes by most people is to break down fats (lipase enzymes), proteins (protease enzyme), carbohydrates (amylase enzyme), and lactose (lactase enzyme), etc. Dipeptidyl dipeptidase IV (DPP-IV) is another enzyme added to many enzyme formulas that helps breaks down gluten, casein, and soy. This enzyme breaks these proteins down into their amino acids to prevent IgG reactions and the formation of caseomorphins and gliadinomorphins from the peptides. DPP-IV is released by intestinal cells and produced by lactic acid bacteria such as those found in yogurt. DPP-IV is able to break down part of the protein in gluten and casein and the opiates created by them. However, DPP IV needs other protease enzymes to complete the job, so most companies make a formula (Houston Enzymes, Kirkman, Enzymedica, and Klaire Labs) with multiple protease enzymes along with DPP-IV. DPP-IV is often in low supply in children with autism. This is true for several reasons: when the gut is injured the intestinal cells can't release DPP IV, excessive mucous from a damaged gut prevents contact with food, and mercury damages the production of this enzyme. Remember that zinc inactivates DPP-IV, and should be taken away from any enzyme formulation containing it.

Enzymes also appear to help with phenols and salicylates for some individuals. One particular company, Houston Nutraceuticals, makes an enzyme called No-Fenol that contains xylanase, which breaks down the cell wall of complex carbohydrates. Dr. Houston has also seen that it helps with yeast conditions in the body. No one is exactly sure how it works but it seems to be effective for many at reducing phenol reactions.

The most common enzymes on the market are plant-based (actually fungal-based), and the type I most often recommend. Choose a high quality plant-based enzyme as they work in a greater pH range and will be able to work both in the stomach and intestinal tract. Pancreatic enzymes, called pancreatin, are from animal sources, typically pigs, and do not survive the acid environment of the stomach; therefore plant-based enzymes are more effective. However, if there is a reaction to the plant enzymes most commonly from a fungal sensitivity, pancreatic enzymes are a good alternative. Fruit enzymes such as bromelain from pineapple and papain from papaya are beneficial enzymes as well although some people are sensitive to the salicylates in them. I find the plant-based to work well for most people.

Enzymes are helpful regardless of diet. They help to breakdown the foods you eat, but do not take the place of special diet. However, enzymes can be useful when a strict diet, for example a gluten and casein-free diet, cannot be observed, or when someone is just transitioning to a diet. While some feel you can take enzymes instead of a special diet, such as GFCF, I have not found this to be true. Also, with celiac disease enzymes cannot be used in place of removing gluten.

If you notice any negative reaction from the enzymes, stop them and slowly introduce them at a fraction of the normal dose. The cleaning up of debris in the gut can expose fresh, sensitive tissue, yeast die-off can cause symptoms, the removal of opiates and other endorphins and brain chemicals from the removal of toxic foods can produce drug withdrawal-like reactions like irritability and hyperactivity. While these may be uncomfortable for the short-term, they are not usually bad for the individual and typically subside in one to two weeks. They usually include symptoms such as stomachache, hyperactivity, flu-like symptoms, or loose bowel movements. If symptoms are strong or continue past a couple weeks, consult a professional.

Take enzymes with the first bite of food or twenty minutes before food if you are using capsules to ensure the breakdown of the capsule ahead of time. If you are taking probiotics too some feel it is important to take them away from each other. I don't know if this is necessary but to be conservative, I suggest taking the probiotics at the end of the meal. For those who can't swallow pills, sprinkle the enzymes on the first few bits of food to make sure they get in. Wash enzymes down with water because the proteases can eat away the dead cells of the mouth exposing fresh skin and this can cause irritation. You can also give enzymes in water or juice. The amount of enzymes to take depends on the size of the meal and the formulation—enzymes are dosed based on the size of the meal rather than the age or weight of the individual.

For much more detailed information on the uses and benefits of enzymes and implementing them, I suggest reading one of Karen DeFelice's books on enzymes, consulting her website www.enzymestuff.com, or joining http://health.groups.yahoo.com/group/EnzymesandAutism/.

Probiotics

Probiotics are beneficial bacteria. There are hundreds of strains in our body and ten times as many good bacteria as cells in our bodies. Technically, we are ten times more bacteria than human; as such we have evolved to live synergistically. Some of the functions of probiotics include:

- Regulate peristalsis and bowel movements.
- Break down bacterial toxins.
- Make vitamins needed and utilized: B1, B2, B3, B5, B6, B12, A and K.
- Digest protein into amino acids (for use by the body).
- Produce antibiotics and antifungals.
- Help breakdown sugars, lactose, and oxalates.
- Support immune system and increase number of immune cells.
- Promote Th-1 immunity and balance Th-2 skewed immunity.
- Balance intestinal pH.
- Protect against environmental toxins: mercury, pesticides, and pollution.

Probiotics are one of my favorite supplements as so many children with ASD have dysbiosis and good bacteria have so many important functions in the body. Find a supplement with multiple strains—both lactobacillus (such as lactobacillus acidophilus in yogurt) and bifido (bifidobacterium longum) strains. Bifidobacterium infantis is present in high amounts in infants. Lactobacillus GG (in Culturelle) is beneficial against clostridia. There are also strains of other microorganisms such as saccharomyces boulardii, a yeast that kills candida, that you can find in some formulations.

For most children on the spectrum who are casein sensitive, make sure to buy a probiotic that does not contain milk. If a child shows regression with probiotics I often find it is due to a yeast overgrowth. As the good bacteria begin to crowd out the yeast, it can produce a die-off and uncomfortable symptoms. Some suggestions for purchasing probiotics:

- Any high quality probiotic containing Lactobacillus acidophilus, Lactobacillus rhamnosis, Lactobacillus G-G, Lactobacillus Longum, Bifidobacter, streptococcus thermophilus) (Pangborn and Baker, 2001).
- Klaire Labs: Therabiotic Complete, Therabiotic Detox (www.klairelabs.com).
- Kirkman Labs: Super Pro-Bio Gold (www.kirkmanlabs.com).
- Custom Probiotics brand is one of the few without SCD illegal fillers such as inulin (www.customprobiotics.com).
- ThreeLac: Helpful for yeast overgrowth (www.globalhealthtrax.com).
- VSL3: contains 450 Billion bacteria (www.vsl3.com).
- Primal Defense: start with 1/2 scoop or 1/2 capsule daily, every two weeks increase dose by 1/2 scoop or 1/2 capsule until 6 scoops or capsules are reached. Continue 6 scoops/capsules for 90 days (www.GardenofLife.com).
- Lactobacillus GG, also known as Culturelle, by VRP (www.lactobacillusgg.com).

Also, fermented foods are rich in probiotics. Kefir, raw sauerkraut, and kombucha are a few that are or can be made non-dairy if necessary. See more on fermented foods in Part 3, Step #7, *Evolve Diet: Nutrition Boosters*.

Butyric Acid

Butyric acid is an important energy source for the cells lining the colon. Butyric acid seems to reduce chronic inflammatory conditions of the colon. It has also been helpful for children with chronic constipation, especially those with large, hard clay-like bowel movements.

Butyric acid works by:
- Reducing the inflammatory condition of these walls reducing intracellular seepage of undigested food particles.
- Sealing up the "holes" left by candida albicans overgrowth that has burrowed into the intestines.
- Stimulating epithelial sloughing in the intestinal tract to help re-establish the balance of beneficial bacteria

It comes in the form of calcium butyrate and magnesium butyrate. Beware though, it has a very strong smell and may be difficult to administer. Some moms have said freezing it makes it smell less.

Additional Supplements

Colostrum

Colostrum is the first fluid (not milk) secreted from the breast of mammals in the initial period after birth before build up of proper flora in the gut in the baby. According to Beth Ley Ph.D., many studies have been done on the ability of colostrum to improve diarrhea in infants and children from nine months to three years (Ley, 2000:54). Colostrum also aids immune function by providing rich immune factors, such as immunoglobulins, antibody-stimulating factors, polypeptides, and many more. Colostrum protects, activates, regulates and supports our immune system (Ley, 2000:69).

For those who are not breast fed: one drop of colostrum per day in formula is recommended for newborns to six months of age, two drops per day in formula for those six months to one year, and three drops per day for those over one year old. It can also be supplemented in older children with poor immune function or diarrhea. Be sure to find a casein-free form if intolerant to casein and an organic source.

Kirkman Labs has a dairy-free form (from cows raised hormone-, pesticide- and antibiotic-free) called Colostrum Gold.

Transfer Factors

Transfer factors are small molecules that consist of specific sequences of amino acids found in colostrum, found in the first milk from the mother that builds the immune system. Transfer factors are not species specific so we can get transfer factor from cows. Transfer factor is typically casein-free. There are antigen specific transfer factors that go after fungi (such as candida) and viruses (such as herpes). Hugh Fudenberg, M.D. conducted a pilot study on transfer factor (dialysable lymphocyte extract) on infantile autism and found it to help 21 out of 22 autistic children, and while five regressed after leaving the treatment, they did not go down to base level (Fudenberg, 1996). Advanced Medical Labs make a candida specific transfer factor.

Phosphatidylcholine

Phosphatidylcholine acts as an important methyl donor but choline also has many important properties. Phosphatidylcholine is the main ingredient in lecithin from egg yolk and soybean. It's the precursor to the neurotransmitter acetylcholine, crucial for thought and memory. Phosphatidylcholine produces myelin for coating nerve and brain cell connections. It aids the functioning of cell membranes to allow nutrients in and toxins out. It also helps protects the liver and helps with brain function including with bipolar disorder.

Medicinal Mushrooms

Medicinal mushrooms have similar immune systems to humans and so they create many wonderful substances that defend us against disease. Maitake, Shiitake, and Reishi all have anti-bacteria, anti-viral and anti-candida properties, as well as immune enhancement properties. Shiitake is a kidney and liver tonic.

People and practitioners often steer away from medicinal mushrooms as they are fungi, which are strictly eliminated on anti-yeast diets because culinary mushrooms (also fungi) are known to aggravate or feed candida. In the case of medicinal mushrooms, this avoidance is not necessary according to Paul Stamets, one of the world's leading mycologists—in fact, medicinal mushrooms kill candida (Stamets lecture, Berkeley, CA, 2002). Gary Null references a study by K. Aduchi which states, "[Maitake] was found to directly activate various effector cells that attack foreign cells (macrophages, natural killer cells...T cells, etc.). and potentiate the activities of various mediators, including lymphokines and interleukin-1" (Null, 2002:534).

There are many formulas and products out there. McCandless recommends Myco-Immune by Thorne, a blend of seven mushrooms for the immune system. Liver Life by BioRay contains several mushrooms and is a great product for liver and detoxification support. New Chapter has some products made Paul Stamets, a world leader in medicinal mushrooms.

Glyconutrients

There are eight glyconutrients in nature but because of our agricultural practices only one, glucose, is still available and prevalent. The eight glyconutrients are: mannose, galactose, glucose, fucose, xylose, n-acetylglucosamine, n-acetylgalactosamine, and n-acetylneuraminic acid.

All necessary glyconutrients and phytonutrients we need for health are deposited only in the final hours or days of ripening on the vine. But almost all produce today is harvested green—picked before it's ripened and shipped to stores to retain shelf life. Some ripen on the way, and others are "gassed" to ripen them.

Because of these practices, we get virtually none of these glyconutrients. Glyconutrients appear to boost immune function, support detoxification, and aid attention and learning. This is an exciting new area of study.

N- acetylglucosamine (NAG), one of the eight glyconutrients, has been found to bind to lectins, neutralizing them. This individual glyconutrient is being tried by some families as an inexpensive way to address lectins.

Coenzyme Q-10 (CoQ10)

CoQ10 is also called ubiquinone, as it is so ubiquitous in every cell of the body. It is used by the mitochondria, where energy is produced in the cell, and a deficiency creates lethargy. CoQ10 deficiency puts stress on the areas that are most metabolically active, such as the muscles, heart, and immune system organs. Stress on the immune system can deplete CoQ10.

Bock most frequently uses it with kids with immune system problems, hypotonia, lethargy, and mitochondrial dysfunction in doses of 30-200 mg per day depending on the form of CoQ10, age and size of child (Bock, 2007).

Pycnogenol

Pycnogenol is a powerful antioxidant that reduces inflammation very effectively. Bock states that it is "one of only a few antioxidants that can cross the blood-brain barrier, and directly enter neurons." Be aware pycnogenol is often made from pine bark extract, a strong phenol. Bock recommends 25-200 mg per day (Bock 2007).

Electrolytes

Electrolytes, also known as ionic solutions, are substances that dissolve in water to provide a solution that conducts an electrical current. Ions of electrolytes are sodium, potassium, calcium, magnesium, chloride, phosphate, and hydrogen carbonate (HCO3-) also know as bicarbonate. Electrolytes alkalize the gut, regulate hydration, influence blood pH, and are critical for nerves, heart, lungs, and muscles as they provide the "electrical signal." KTS makes several proprietary solutions called Peltier Electrolytes™ (www.kt-solutions.com).

Sulfates

As discovered by Waring, up to 92% of children with autism have a problem with sulfation. They are not able to utilize the sulfates they ingest, and in fact, the sulfates they so desperately need may cause distress. Waring has not done research as to whether certain sulfates taken orally can be utilized by these individuals better than others. Lang has had experience with supplementing with sulfates orally and has seen positive results with his own children and clients. For this reason, I believe sulfates could be very beneficial for individuals with faulty sulfation by providing the body with the building block needed to support proper sulfate-dependant processes including digestion, detoxification, membrane/tissue repair, and intestinal integrity. One of the best ways to supplement sulfate is with Epsom salts, the common name for magnesium sulfate. It appears to absorb and be utilized well. There are differing opinions on whether supplementing sulfate orally is effective. According to Lang, oral sulfates that appear to be beneficial without causing problems for most children include: methylsulfonylmethane, biotin, thiamin, N-Acetyl Cysteine (NAC), glucosamine sulfate, N-Acetyl Glucosamine and bromelain (Lang, 2002). Lang's company, BrainChild Nutritionals, makes Intestimend, a product with many of these sulfates. For each of these, doses are best divided and given throughout the day and are based on a 50-pound child.

Similarly to cysteine (a substance rich in sulfate that is often not well tolerated), some children cannot tolerate sulfur-rich foods. However, if tolerated, consider adding these sulfur-containing foods: cruciferous vegetables such as broccoli, cabbage (raw sauerkraut is a good source), cauliflower, brussel sprouts, garlic, onions, and eggs.

Interesting note: Sometime I see the whole family of sulfur-rich foods (onions, garlic, shallots, leeks, cabbage, eggs, dairy and whey products, bok choy, cauliflower, broccoli, brussel sprouts, kale, turnips, and asparagus) causing problems for those with ASD. It would seem to make sense that if you are low in sulfur, eat sulfur rich foods. However, these foods often cause digestive disturbances (which I suppose could be many things: sulfur feeding yeast, difficult to digest, etc), and more strangely sometimes show up as reactive on IgG panels. Andrew Cutler, Ph.D, talks about this in more detail in his book *Amalgam Illness*.

DMAE

DMAE is a neurotransmitter precursor that, according to Block helps to improve behaviors, mental concentration, puzzle solving ability and organization and had been reported in the *Journal of Pediatrics* back in 1958,. DMAE is recommended by Dr. Mary Ann Block for autism (Block, 2002).

However, according to Dr. Walsh, some children can benefit from while others should avoid DMAE. During his work with metallothionein dysfunction with autism, he states "45% of our autistic population exhibit undermethylation which can be effectively treated with supplements of methionine, magnesium, DMG, SAM(e), and calcium, along with strict avoidance of DMAE and folic acid. In contrast, 15% of people with autism exhibit over methylation and benefit from liberal doses of DMAE, folic acid, and B12, along with strict avoidance of methionine and SAM(e)" (McCandless, 2004). SAM has a fairly poor parent rating according to ARI publication 34.

Therefore, I do not suggest DMAE as a blanket recommendation; however, a trial may helpful as long as symptomology and behavior are closely monitored. Additionally, the Bioenergy Balancing Center (See *Additional Author Comments*) feels that DMAE assisting in detoxifying the body of fluoride.

5-HTP (5-hydroxytryptophan)

5-HTP is the precursor to serotonin, which then converts to melatonin. It is often quite effective for depression. I use this one more with adults. If depression is present, after you consider adrenal and thyroid function, consider an inability to make or methylate neurotransmitters such as serotonin. 5-HTP is one way to address this low serotonin. Do not use 5-HTP with medications that address serotonin (such as SSRIs) without the supervision of a physician.

Adrenal Extract or Glandular

Adrenal extracts are dried and ground adrenal gland typically from beef sources. Adrenal cortex extract is just the cortex versus the whole gland. Adrenal cortex is better at normalizing cortisol levels. This supplement can support the adrenals, and can boost energy, reduce the effects of stress, and reduce inflammation. This supplement can be helpful for adrenal fatigue and excess cortisol levels. Thorne Research makes an adrenal cortex product.

Lectin Lock and NAG

Lectin Lock is a supplement being used by parents whose children have problems with lectins. It is a blend of supplements that bind to the lectins, preventing them from causing damage. Bladderwrack, okra, and d-mannose are some of the ingredients. D-mannose is an essential sugar that binds to lectins. N-acetylglucosamine (NAG), the most abundant ingredient, binds specifically to the wheat lectin, wheat germ agglutinin (WGA). Some parents have been trying NAG only with success. Find more information at: relentlessimprovement.com/catalog/lectin-lock.htm and http://health.groups.yahoo.com/group/lectins_in_autism/.

Melatonin

Melatonin is the hormone that regulates sleep. Supplementation with melatonin has been found to support children with ASD with sleep challenges. It is helpful for falling asleep, nighttime waking, and early morning waking. Melatonin is also an antioxidant for the brain.

As it's a hormone, one holistically-oriented physician suggests it's best for short-term use (three months or less), and best to rule out other causes of sleep issues, and try other alternatives such as keeping the room dark or homeopathic sleep remedies. Ross recommends not using melatonin with children. However, many parents use melatonin, it has been reported to help 61% of children and according to ARI; 'Melatonin seems to be exceptionally safe, and high dosages in animals produce no toxicity" (Adams, 2007). Bock suggests between .5 to 3 mg of melatonin at night (Bock 2007).

Herbs

Brainchild Nutritionals put together a wonderful paper on their Herbathione product, which uses the following herbs to aid in detoxification and a host of other functions (from www.brainchildnutritionals.com, reprinted with permission).

- **Ashwaganda** supports detoxification via its antioxidant function in the recycling of glutathione and support of superoxide dismutase. It is also a nervous system rejuvenator/protectant, for immune support, and for support of sleep disturbances, wasting diseases, failure to thrive in children, joint and nerve pains.

- **Burdock Root** promotes bile flow, liver cleansing, and enhanced liver glutathione. It is a blood cleanser and purifier, used with inflammatory conditions of chronic toxicity and for skin conditions. It reduces inflammation, is a mild laxative, and controls bacterial infection. Burdock supports lung, kidney, spleen, pituitary, lymphatic, thymus, and immune health.

- **Astragalus Root** is a nourishing tonic that stimulates the immune system, spleen, lungs, adrenals, liver, circulator, lymphatic, and urinary systems, lowers blood pressure and blood sugar levels. Aids digestion, promotes healing, inhibits lipid peroxidation.

- **Fennel Seed** promotes gastrointestinal motility, the functions of the liver, kidneys, spleen and supports respiratory function. It relieves abdominal pain, colon disorders, gas, and gastrointestinal tract spasms. It is also a natural sulfur source.

- **Ginkgo Biloba** increases cellular glutathione and liver-specific glutathione S-transferase. It is a powerful antioxidant, dilates bronchial tubes and blood vessels, specifically increases cerebral and cardiac blood flow and available cerebral oxygen, controls allergic responses, and improves cardio-pulmonary function. It has anti-fungal and antibacterial effects. Ginkgo is used for asthma, allergic inflammatory responses, cerebral insufficiency, and depression. It inhibits allergic response and improves digestion.

- **Gotu Kola** is a potent antioxidant, it can raise levels of glutathione and antioxidant enzymes including catalase, glutathione peroxidase and superoxide dismutase. It improves circulatory problems in the extremities and speeds healing. Gotu kola is a rejuvenating herb that helps in wound healing, ulcerative conditions, depression and other nervous disorders. Improves muscle tone and cardio-pulmonary function. It also normalizes blood pH.

- **Milk Thistle** protects the liver against toxins, particularly lipid peroxidation. Herbal antioxidant/free radical quencher. Leukotriene inhibitor. Helps to detoxify alcohol, drugs, and other chemical toxins. It regenerates liver cells and stimulates bile flow, relaxes spasms, and is a sulfur source. Assists in regeneration of glutathione and restoration of cellular thiol status. Kidney support. Adrenal support. Aids inflammatory bowel disorders, weakened immune function.

- **Sarsaparilla** clears toxins, particularly mercury and other heavy metals, and supports the liver, and urinary tract. Enhances activities of antioxidant enzymes catalase, superoxide dismutase, and glutathione peroxidase.

- **Schisandra** supports detoxification via recycling of glutathione and is a liver protectant. It acts as a tonic for the nervous, urinary, and cardiac systems. Schisandra is traditionally used for asthma, night sweats, urinary disorders, chronic and early morning diarrhea, palpitations, insomnia, poor memory.

Salt

While salt is not a "supplement" in our normal definition, it is a very important substance to discuss. Salt is not the terrible substance we always hear negative things about. Stripped down sodium chloride—that is, common table salt—may be, but natural salt is much different.

Salt is essential for life. The crystalline structure of salt is electric not molecular. Salt conducts the electrical system of the body, which allows the nervous system, heart, and lungs to function. Without salt, we could not think or function. Good quality salt has minerals, and while it does not contain vitamins or proteins, salt with water and light can create highly geometrical structures biochemically identical to vitamins and proteins (Hendel, 2003:99).

I have found many, if not most, children I see in my practice with autistic spectrum disorders crave salt. I believe this is because they are deficient and craving minerals. Out of the 94 natural elements of the periodic table, crystal salt contains all of them with the exception of the inert gases. While our body is craving these minerals it is looking for in the salt most of us consume stripped table salt with none of the minerals we are missing, so the cravings continue.

Table salt, as I mentioned, is not healthful. It is completely devoid of any micronutrients except the bare minimum—sodium and chloride—and is depleting as a substance. Sea salt is much better, but be sure you use the naturally evaporated salt, not the stripped, bleached sea salt. Celtic salt is popular among the DAN! practitioners, and it's an even better option than sea salt. However, crystal salt is the best. It contains the highest number of trace and nutritive minerals and has a crystalline structure that has beneficial energetic properties. I use is Himalayan Crystal Salt that I get at americanbluegreen.com.

So if your child craves salt, do not hold back on it, but use a high quality Celtic or crystal salt. There is a great book called *Water and Salt: The Essence of Life* by Hendel and Ferreira, if you are interested in learning more about this subject.

ASD Diet Options

As you may have found out already, there are many diet protocols used with ASD. It can be very confusing and difficult to sort out all of the information, to know which diet or diets best suit your situation, and how strictly you need to implement it or them. Often parents do a great job implementing GFCF but when it comes to integrating GFCF with a yeast protocol and low phenols, things can get confusing. The following table lists some details of the diets, when they tend to be most effective, some of the pitfalls for implementing them, and when you need to follow them strictly. These basic summaries can help you determine which diet might be right for your particular needs and help you navigate implementation. The details of each diet are described below this section.

I divide diets into two categories; Foundational diets (diets parents often start with) and Layering diets (diets to layer onto, refine, and customize). Any diet can be a foundational diet. I chose the following because they are often the most popular, effective, and straightforward to start with. However, any diet can be implemented at any time, and in any order or combination.

Overview of Diet Options

	Diet	When to Use/Strictness	Benefits	Pitfalls/Disadvantages
Foundational Diets	**GFCF** No gluten or casein.	Good starting point. Must follow strictly.	Fairly easy to do once you get the hang of it. According to ARI survey of parents, 65% of those with ASD receive benefit.	Enzymes do not help for all people. Often substitute with a lot of sugar.
	SCD (Specific Carbohydrate Diet) Restricts carbohydrates to only fruits, non-starchy vegetables, and honey. No grains, starchy vegetables, or mucilaginous fibers.	Typically great for those with yeast overgrowth, bacterial imbalance, gut inflammation, and chronic diarrhea. Must follow strictly.	Allows for sweet foods typically not allowed on anti-yeast diets such as honey and fruit. 66% of parents reported benefit from SCD	Difficult to follow for some very picky eaters. Nuts are relied on heavily and more difficult for those with nut allergies. May help or may be problematic with constipation.
	Body Ecology Diet Anti-yeast diet combining principles of anti-yeast diets including no sugar, acid/alkaline, fermented foods, etc.	For yeast overgrowth. Will want to avoid sugar – but not strictly avoid any molecule of sugar.	Very comprehensive. Works well on yeast overgrowth. 55% of parents reported benefit from a candida diet.	Combines many principles that may be confusing or challenging.
	Nourishing Traditions/ Weston A. Price Diet	Use with almost everyone for brain nourishment and digestion.	Very nourishing. Solid nutrition principles. Easy to digest. Healthy fermented foods.	High fat is problematic for some.

Layering ASD Diets

	Diet	When to Use/Strictness	Benefits	Pitfalls/Disadvantages
Refining and Layering/Customizing the Diet	**Food Sensitivities** Eliminating all food sensitivities.	One of the important first steps. Depending – may need to be strict or rotate foods.	Essential step that often improves digestion, attention and learning, and reduces allergies and pain. Once you know *what* foods to remove, doing so it not difficult (depending on the foods).	Can be difficult to identify offending foods, and if many foods are positive on testing, options can become limited. Rotation diets can be complicated.
	Elimination Diet	To determine food sensitivities. Short term "testing" diet	Best way to determine food sensitivities.	Sometimes it can be difficult to determine reactions from foods in some children.
	Rotation Diet	When food sensitivities are mild and tolerated on a limited basis. Can be strictly followed but often more flexibility allowed.	Provides flexibility by allowing consumption of additional foods. 50% of parents reported benefit.	Determining whether a food is tolerated on a limited basis or not at all.
	Feingold Diet/Phenol Protocol Restricts high phenolic foods, including all artificial ingredients and many fruits.	For those with phenolic reactions: red cheeks, ears, hyperactivity, lethargy, inappropriate laughter, reactions to artificial ingredients. Can not be "phenol-free" – no "strict adherence."	Highly beneficial and fairly easy to implement. 55% of parents reported benefit.	Few pitfalls. No test for phenol sensitivity.
	Low Oxalate Diet Restricts high oxalate foods, includes supplementation of calcium, probiotics, and other nutrients.	For urinary, GI or other pain, craving high oxalate food, continued constipation, diarrhea, or gas not relieved by other diets. Poor growth can be due to oxalates. Can add a limited amount of oxalates – no "strict adherence."	Seems to be a missing piece for those who have tried GFCF, SCD, and other diets with only moderate success.	Fairy new diet with not a lot of clinical data. A new hypothesis suggests vitamin K deficiency may be involved and correcting this may make this diet unnecessary. Reduces vitamin C because it can convert to oxalates.

Layering ASD Diets

	Diet	When to Use/Strictness	Benefits	Pitfalls/Disadvantages
Refining and Layering/Customizing the Diet	**Feast Without Yeast** Standard anti-yeast diet with no sugar, yeast foods, etc.	For yeast overgrowth. Will want to avoid sugar – but not strictly avoid any molecule of sugar.	Works well for yeast overgrowth. 55% of parents reported benefit from a candida diet.	No sugars allowed which can be challenging.
	Raw Food Diet Eat all or some raw foods to take burden off pancreas.	For digestion, acid/alkaline balance, and in warm weather. Not need to follow strictly.	A 100% raw diet has been very effective for a small group. However, better to incorporate some raw foods into other diet.	Raw foods are not easy for everyone to digest, not good for "cold/damp" conditions like candida.
	Paleolithic Diet	Helpful for those who can't eat grains or have blood sugar regulation and digestion problems.	Similar to SCD, maybe a bit less restrictive.	Difficult for a child that does not eat meat and/or vegetables.
	GAPS Diet (Gut and Psychology Syndrome)	This diet is essentially SCD.	See SCD	See SCD
	Ketogenic diet	A diet for seizures, when all other options are exhausted.	Has good success helping the more severe seizure disorders.	Requires medical supervision. Very restrictive. Unable to meet nutrition needs without supplementation

Gluten- and Casein-Free Diet (GFCF)

I recommend most people try GFCF regardless of the IgG and opiate test results. The test results can be incorrect and so many children show some level of improvement that the diet is worth the effort. Some DAN! physicians require their patients to be on the GFCF diet before they will see someone in their practice. Other physicians feel it is really important to test for celiac before starting the diet so an accurate diagnosis can be determined.

Gluten is the protein found in wheat, rye, barley, commercial oats (there are special gluten-free oats you can order online, glutenfreeoats.com), kamut, and spelt. Casein is the protein found in dairy. There are dozens if not hundreds of hidden sources of gluten. It is important to do this diet correctly because any small infraction can make the diet ineffective. Read a book, join an online chat group, and/or work with a doctor or nutrition consultant to learn the nuances (more in *Resources* section).

Common symptoms of gluten/casein intolerance: The same symptoms of intolerance for food sensitivities apply here. Where gluten and other food sensitivities typically cause diarrhea or constipation, casein intolerance is most often associated with significant constipation. Additionally, vomiting clear mucus and leg aches or "growing pains" are most commonly a sign of casein sensitivity. Fuzzy thinking, high pain tolerance, self-injurious behavior and other common opiate symptoms are associated with gluten and casein intolerance.

When to use this diet: I recommend this as a starting point or foundation for most diets. If you choose to begin with another diet, I would recommend that this diet be gluten- and casein-free as well. For instance, if you do SCD I would not recommend including cheese and yogurt which is allowed on an SCD diet, until you are confident these foods are not a problem. GFCF often improves symptoms of constipation and diarrhea. It also reduces many cognitive and behavioral symptoms for many children.

Pitfalls: There are so many hidden sources of gluten and even casein that it can be difficult to eliminate all infractions, and it is essential to do so to see if the diet is effective. Also, GFCF foods are not necessarily healthy foods. There are many GFCF cookies, crackers, candy, cakes that are loaded with sugar. Be sure to implement a low sugar version of the GFCF diet. If you need to just substitute food for food (as an example, the gluten-free waffle for the regular waffle) at first during the withdrawal phase and reduce sugar later, that is fine for the short term. However, don't get complacent about leaving sugar in the diet. Also, be careful of corn and soy as wheat and dairy substitutes—these are common food sensitivities for many.

When dairy and wheat are removed from the diet, many helpful nutrients and properties are lost. Dairy (particularly raw dairy) has been found to reduce risk of asthma in children. Butter and raw butter contain butyric acid, which nourishes the brain and intestinal lining and has antimicrobial properties. Dairy is rich in methionine, an important amino acid for methylation. Of course, dairy is a good source of calcium (a calcium supplement is important with a GFCF diet). See Calcium in Impact of Nutrients for non-dairy sources of calcium. Whey (a protein in dairy) is rich in the precursor to glutathione (cysteine), lactoferrin, immunoglobin and growth factors. Fermented dairy is a wonderful way to get probiotics. When dairy is removed, hydrogenated margarine and other unhealthy oils are sometimes substituted adding junk to the diet. Whole wheat has a high level of fiber and phosphorus, a moderate level of protein, thiamine, magnesium, and iron, and even a small amount of methionine. When a GFCF diet is implemented, these helpful nutrients and properties can be difficult to obtain.

Clinical experience: One two and a half year old boy went from zero words to over 200 in 3 months of GFCF. Many parents report their child will expand their very narrow food choices once the addicting opiates (gluten and casein) are removed—one child starting eating vegetables for the first time, a couple others started eating meat. Many therapists and learning specialists notice the child is paying attention and learning much better (and asking the parents what they changed). Digestion is often one of the biggest areas to improve—constipation is eliminated when dairy is removed, diarrhea goes away when gluten is removed, gas and pain are reduced or eliminated.

See Appendix V for information on implementing a GFCF diet.

Specific Carbohydrate Diet (SCD)

The Specific Carbohydrate Diet introduced by Dr. Merrill Haas and made popular by Elaine Gottschall in *Breaking the Vicious Cycle: Intestinal Health Through Diet* eliminates all disaccharides (two-sugar molecules) and polysaccharides (starches). Only monosaccharides (glucose, fructose and galactose) such as fruits, honey, and most non-starchy vegetables are allowed. In a nutshell (so to speak), this means all sugars (except monosaccharides) and starches are out, including but not limited to table sugar, maple syrup, rice, pastas, breads, potatoes, certain beans, rice milk, and cornstarch.

The diet uses the principle that some individuals cannot digest carbohydrates, most likely due to damage to the small intestine mucosa. This maldigestion leads to malabsorption of disaccharides, which cause bacteria and yeast overgrowth as they feed on the unabsorbed complex sugars. These bacteria destroy enzymes further inhibiting carbohydrate metabolism and creating further damage to the small intestine villi and microvilli completing a "vicious cycle" that continues to deteriorate.

Since monosaccharides are already single sugar molecules nothing needs to be broken down. By absorbing immediately into the small intestine, these sugars can be eaten with no problem and appear to not feed the harmful microorganisms.

Some comments on dairy and raw dairy

Please note that SCD allows for dairy that is lactose free, including certain cheeses and homemade yogurt. Those individuals with casein sensitivity should not include dairy products. However, some researchers and clinicians such as Dr. Mercola (www.mercola.com) believe that the problems with dairy stem from pasteurization, as this process kills the natural enzymes and good bacteria found naturally in milk. It is hypothesized that pasteurization (and maybe homogenization) changes the molecular structure of the protein molecules possibly causing casein intolerance. Additionally, commercial milk is from cows fed grain rather than grass-fed, which could be creating the inflammation found in those who are sensitive to dairy. Some clients of mine, once they spent time healing the gut, were able to consume raw dairy. In one study, Lactobacillus rhamnosus GG reduced casein sensitivity in infants (Isolaruri, 2001). Perhaps, as the gut heals and good bacteria are restored, dairy can be consumed without inflammatory reaction. Raw dairy contains good bacteria, enzymes, and butyric acid which helps support a healthy intestinal tract. Some states ban the sale of raw dairy and people wishing to obtain it must participate in a cow share program. Other people buy raw milk as "pet food" from their state or another state (Organic Pastures from California does so). Based on my personal experience of using raw yogurt, my clients' experience with raw dairy, and the research I have done I feel comfortable with raw dairy. However, many scary things have been said about raw dairy, especially for those who are immune-compromised, so in order to be comfortable with your decision and other people's responses do your own research before proceeding on this personal decision.

See Appendix VIII for more details on raw dairy. There is more information on my website (NourishingHope.com), and well as on RealMilk.com.

When to use this diet: SCD was originally used for those with severe intestinal damage suffering from diseases like ulcerative colitis, Crohn's, and celiac. It can be very help for those with ASD that involve chronic diarrhea. While some practitioners use SCD for those with "simple" candida overgrowth; I prefer to use it for those with candida that have diarrhea and/or chronic inflammation. For other cases of candida, I typically use other diets—as this diet can be difficult for some and I'm not completely convinced that the yeast is not fed by the monosaccharides. For this diet to work, no infractions may occur so while you can add further restrictions to it (for example, eliminating dairy), you cannot add "illegal" foods to the diet.

Pitfalls: As this diet does not use any starches, nut flours are highly relied on for making "crackers" and "breads." This makes it very difficult for those with nut allergies and intolerances or schools that have a no nut policy. It can be done without nuts but the child needs to have a diverse enough diet to eat basically meat, vegetables, and fruit. Too high protein is also a concern on this diet, as it can create high ammonia in the body. If someone eats a lot of (SCD-compliant) beans, oxalates and lectins can be a problem for some.

Clinical Experience: Some children have a wonderful response to this diet. A smaller percentage of my clients are on this diet compared to GFCF but for those that it works for, it works amazingly well. Children often have diarrhea go away on this diet. I've heard several stories from parents at conferences that for some children with chronic inflammation, who are on steroids, this diet has been literally a lifesaver. In my practice, I find that this diet works wonders in a short period of time (couple days to a couple weeks), if it's going to work.

See Appendix IX for more information on implementing SCD.

The Body Ecology Diet

The Body Ecology Diet incorporates excellent principles of proper food combining, acid/alkaline balance with low acid-forming foods, low/no sugars and starches, easily digestible foods, fermented foods, and other solid nutrition recommendations to clear up candida overgrowth in the body. The diet allows a few grains such as quinoa, millet buckwheat, and amaranth when properly soaked.

Acid/alkaline is the principle of eating mostly alkaline forming foods. This will assist the body in maintaining a slightly alkaline blood pH. When the body is too acidic it leaches alkalizing mineral from the bones to balance the pH. Alkalizing the system supports the health of the gut as well. The standard American diet is awfully acid forming: sugar, meat, processed foods, and refined grains and carbohydrates. As meat is acid-forming, this diet uses much less animal protein than the SCD and others. The most alkalizing foods are most mineral rich so vegetables top the list. The particular grains that are allowed are on the alkalizing side, while rice, wheat, oats, and most others are acid-forming. Note that acid-forming foods are not necessarily acidic foods; for example, while lemons are acidic, they are alkalizing (creating an alkaline ash in the body).

When to use this diet: The Body Ecology Diet is great for clearing up candida overgrowth. It goes a step further than anti-candida diets that simply restrict sugars, and fermented/moldy foods.

Pitfalls: This diet requires proper food combining. If someone has very limited or no consumption of vegetables this diet can be difficult. Additionally, while some kids like or warm up to cultured vegetables and kefir, it can be challenging to get children to consume these fermented foods. Finally, it combines many principles that can be confusing and require quite a bit of education at first.

Clinical Experience: Several parents in my practice have seen great results with their children from this diet—clearing up the yeast can really improve gas, digestion, and absorption of nutrients benefiting many bodily systems.

See BodyEcologyDiet.com, or the book, *Body Ecology Diet*, by Donna Gates as well as *Resources* in the Appendices.

Nourishing Traditions/Weston A. Price Diet (NT/WAP)

Weston A. Price was a dentist in the 1930s and 40s who was very interested nutrition and health. He studied indigenous cultures around the world before globalization to see whether there was a connection between nutrition and health. He tried to discover what the culture had in common to keep the people healthy. While there were cultures that ranged from mostly plant foods to exclusively animal foods, he did not find an exclusively plant eating (vegan) group. All cultures had learned that the more balanced diets, of some animal and some plant food, were the healthiest.

Sally Fallon popularized Weston A. Price's work with her wonderful book, *Nourishing Traditions*. This diet uses Price's findings as a foundation for healthy eating. As Price lived in the time where food additives and processed foods were just coming into the food supply and before most indigenous cultures were influenced by "modern commerce," he was able see the effects of modern diet versus the traditional cultures' diets. It was an important observation that is not available today. We are very fortunate he observed and recorded this information. This was also a time when farming and animal husbandry animals used natural, sustainable techniques—not used in today's commercial farming. The Weston A. Price foundation and many small family farms are promoting a return to this way of farming and living that supports the health of the animals, the people who eat them, the land, and our future. In addition to producing food of the highest nutritional quality, the Nourishing Traditions/Weston A. Price diet includes a focus on:
   • Animal foods and fats such as eggs, butter and dairy, beef and other animal protein, that are all pasture-raised or grass-fed, and additional saturated fats such as coconut oil. A belief that saturated fat and cholesterol are good for health.
   • Raw, unprocessed dairy products
   • Soaking and sprouting grains, beans and seeds for increased digestibility and nutrient availability
   • Stocks, broths, and nutrient-dense foods
   • Lacto-fermented foods (not a finding of Price but a cultural consistency)

- Avoiding "foods of modern commerce" such as processed foods with additives, soy foods (unless traditionally fermented), and refined sugar.

This diet is high in omega-3, saturated fat (animal fat and coconut oil), and cholesterol—substances that are important to a healthy brain. Often children (and adults) do well with a diet of 40% or more fat. Recommendations like this are unheard of in mainstream nutrition but very helpful for many. Fallon's other book, *Eat Fat Lose Fat*, has great information on coconut oil. Mary Enig's book, *Know Your Fats*, is another great book on fats.

The health benefits of many of these foods can be found in the Holistic Nutrition, Part 3, Step #7, Evolving the Diet: Nutrition Boosters.

When to use this diet: This is a nourishing diet that can be applied to any other diet someone is on. The Nourishing Traditions/WAP diet is great diet for brain, neurotransmitter and cellular function through the introduction of omega-3 and saturated fats. Implement any principles that will work—there is no "strict adherence" to this diet. The WAP diet is a wonderful diet for a pregnant mother.

Pitfalls: This diet is high in fat and can be problematic for those with gall bladder and fat digestion problems.

Clinical Experience: Many parents tell me they feel "nourished" while on this diet. They also report that their children often attend better in school and that the fermented foods aid digestion and reduce sugar cravings. Kids often love some of the fermented drinks such as kombucha and the fermented "sodas." However, I had a colleague who had a gallbladder attack from this diet as it was too high in fat for her.

Food Sensitivities

Removing all food sensitivities is a basic step in the process of cleaning up any diet. Regardless of which diet you choose, removing food sensitivities is crucial. This step is often more of a refinement for other diets, rather than a diet by it self. However, sometimes an individual's main diet problems may "simply" be food sensitivity related and removing the offending foods may be the only changes to the diet.

Sometimes the foods need to be strictly avoided. Other times, small amounts are tolerated and a rotation diet works well. See rotation diets next.

Common symptoms of food sensitivities: Diarrhea and/or constipation, hyperactivity or lethargy, aches and pains, depression, irritability, aggression, restlessness, and tantrums.

When to use this diet: Always remove all food sensitivities. Determine food sensitivities through an Elimination/Provocation diet or laboratory testing. Adapt any diet by removing all food sensitivities.

Pitfalls: There are no real pitfalls to this. It should always be done. The challenge may be in determining which foods are sensitivities and what to do when the child is sensitive to everything. The elimination diet can be restrictive, and the IgG antibody test can provide both false positives and negatives.

Clinical Experience: Removing food sensitivities often clears up a problems dramatically. The main areas affected are digestion and elimination, inflammation and pain, and mood and energy. I've seen diarrhea clear up overnight or within days, constipation significantly improve, the frequency of stomachaches reduce, and irritability and fatigue decrease.

Elimination Diet

The diet is short term "testing diet" that involves eliminating possible problematic foods for one week, including dairy products, wheat, eggs, corn, sugar, chocolate, peanuts, citrus, food colorings, food additives, and preservatives. Then, one food at a time is introduced into the diet by ingesting two servings, one for breakfast, one for lunch, so that by the end of the day at least a normal amount of the food has been eaten. Record the results. If the food is not offending it may be continued through the remainder of the test. A new food is tested every three days. Of course, I would recommend never adding any additives and preservatives back into the diet. It takes about a month (occasionally longer) to complete the elimination and testing phases.

When to use this diet: Use when you are trying to determine what food sensitivities or other food intolerances are present.

Pitfalls: This diet is restrictive for a child. Sometimes parents find it difficult to notice food reactions in their child.

Clinical Experience: While sometimes reactions are clear and obvious, sometimes parents have a very difficult time identifying food reactions. In children where this reaction is clear, it is very easy to determine food sensitivities and problematic foods. However, in quite a few cases, parents have difficulty making this assessment. In these cases I suggest to continue with the diet, do not allow any infractions, and record (in a diet journal) various factors such as school stress, colds, allergies, and other situations that may make reactions confusing. Eventually, most food sensitivities become clear over time.

See Appendix X for more information in implementing an elimination diet to determine food sensitivities.

Rotation Diet

A rotation diet is where you rotate foods to avoid eating the same food every day to prevent a food reaction or food sensitivity from being created. This is often a good idea but it can get complicated. An ideal rotation diet involves rotating foods every three to four days; however, there are times when diets are very restrictive and this is too difficult. In those cases, even avoiding the food for one day and doing an "every other day" rotation is better than nothing.

You can just rotate the problematic food or you can rotate all foods in a food category. For really sensitive people, where we are trying to avoid new sensitivities, rotating foods in a category is the best. Most commonly I rotate grains (for example, rice on Monday and Thursday, corn Tuesday, wild rice Wednesday, quinoa on Friday, buckwheat on Saturday, and amaranth and millet on Sunday. Additionally, I may rotate meats, nuts, and sometimes vegetables. Karyn Seroussi has a good example of a rotation diet in her book *Unraveling the Mystery of Autism and Pervasive Developmental Disorder*.

When to use this diet: A food rotation diet (or rotation diet) is often helpful with food sensitivities where foods cannot be avoided because the diet is limited or when there are such a large number of foods involved.

Pitfalls: It can get complicated and restrictive. Also, there are not eight days in a week so for a strict four day rotation, each week would be different. One week rice would be Monday and Friday, then the next week it's Tuesday and Saturday. There isn't a consistent schedule as with a three day where you can have the food twice in a week and do the same thing every week for ease. For example, every Monday is rice day, Tuesday is corn, and so on.

Clinical Experience: I often use rotation diets in families where rice is a sensitivity and can't be removed completely. On many occasions, this diet allows children to eat a food without a reaction. While keeping it as simple as possible, parents find it an effective way to minimize food reactions.

Feingold Diet and Phenol Protocol

As we have seen in great detail, many individuals with ASD and other neurological and immune system disorders appear to have faulty sulfation and cannot process phenols well. This protocol reduces phenols in the diet. The Phenol Protocol is an approach that I put together that includes several components: 1) a low phenol diet, in most cases, the Feingold Diet, which is a low salicylate diet, 2) supplements and substances that add sulfate to aid sulfation, and 3) enzymes to help break down remaining phenols. There is no way to eliminate 100% of all phenols, so this diet is not an all or nothing program. There are other low phenol diets such as the Failsafe diet, Sarah's diet, Some people may need to be keep phenols very low, while others may only need to reduce phenols by avoiding the high phenol foods such as apples and grapes. This protocol is often used in conjunction with other diets.

The Feingold diet eliminates all artificial phenolic additives and certain salicylates. If you see a discrepancy between a salicylate list (Appendix XI) and Feingold (Appendix XII), it is because Feingold does not eliminate all salicylates, only the ones they have found children (and some adults) to be most reactive to. This means that some foods that have higher salicylate values are allowed on Feingold such as watermelon.

Common symptoms of phenol intolerance: Dark circles under eyes, red face/ears, diarrhea, hyperactivity, impulsivity, aggression, headache, head banging/self-injury, impatience, short attention span, difficulty falling asleep, night waking for several hours, inappropriate laughter, hives, stomach aches, bedwetting and day wetting, dyslexia, speech difficulties, tics, and some forms of seizures.

When to use this diet: Use of these "phenol diets" can be tricky to determine. There is no test to determine faulty sulfation. As I have mentioned, I use several factors to make this determination: 1) reaction to phenolic foods, 2) reaction to Tylenol or acetaminophen and artificial ingredients, 3) levels of sulfate in the blood and urine, 4) test results from phase II liver panel and sulfation capabilities, and 5) family history of neurological disorders including ASD. If self-injurious behavior is present I work with the individual's physician and strongly suggest considering the implementation of a low phenol diet, especially if a GFCF diet has been implemented with no relief.

Pitfalls: At times, these diets can be challenging to implement in conjunction with other diets, because several other diets (especially SCD) limit many foods and rely on fruit for sweets. As fruits are so high in phenols, the limitation of fruits can be very restricting with certain diet combinations.

Clinical Experience: This diet is fairly easy to implement, as it does not remove any food categories completely only certain fruits and vegetables, and particular foods from a food group. The negative food reactions often happen within a short time, around 30 minutes, making it easier to spot reactions. Over time, many of my clients seem to be able to handle more phenols. I assume it is from working on methylation, building up sulfate reserves, reducing the body's burden of toxins, improving digestion and detoxification, and other positive changes that happen over time from supplementation and diet intervention. One or two parents have told me that a diet high in natural food enzymes (a high raw food diet) seemed to allow their child to consume small to moderate amounts of phenols with no reaction. Other parents have reported that phenol intolerance disappeared after chelation. It appears that once you get the system functioning better, phenols are not as much of a problem.

Failsafe and Sarah's Diets are variations of Feingold (see below). While Failsafe is more restrictive, it is very effective for some and really helps reduce migraines and asthma in those chemically sensitive. Sarah's Diet is helpful for some; however, I've had very few clients who have needed this added level of restriction.

Failsafe Diet: Failsafe adds further restrictions to the Feingold Diet by eliminating all high salicylates (not just the "reactive" ones of Feingold), amines, free glutamates, and additional additives and strong smelling foods. Amines can be attached to phenols, salicylates, and other substances and are foods that are frequently associated with migraines. Some of these foods that contain amines include bananas, figs, dates, pork, turkey, chocolate, and cheese. See Appendix XIII for more information on Failsafe.

Sarah's Diet: Sarah's Diet, while not a phenolic diet, also limits fruits and vegetables, in this case those with the carotenoid lutein. You often hear of this as the white food diet as it eliminates most fruits and vegetables with color such as leafy greens, yellow corn, broccoli, green peas, pumpkin, summer (yellow) squash, carrots, brussels sprouts, currants, green olives, green peppers, green beans (pod), plums, peaches, oranges, avocados, and kiwis.

Low Oxalate Diet (LOD)

An oxalate is a salt of oxalic acid that binds to a certain mineral such as calcium, at which point an oxalate crystal is created. Oxalate crystals can be damaging. Normally, a healthy gut will not absorb too many oxalates (naturally occurring in high levels in certain foods) from the diet because as they come through the digestive tract where they are metabolized by the good bacteria in the gut or bind to calcium and are excreted in the stool. However, when the gut is leaky these oxalates are absorbed and high levels end up in the blood, urine, and tissues—especially damaged tissue. Once the oxalates are in the tissue, they create inflammation and pain. This cycle contributes to further inflammation in the intestines and more profound leaky gut. In cells, oxalates can lead to oxidative damage, depletion of glutathione, pain associated with urination, and inflammation related to the immune system.

High oxalate foods - For a more thorough list oxalate foods see Appendix XIV:
- Greens: spinach, Swiss chard, beet greens, parsley.
- Nuts and seeds: almonds, cashews, and peanuts.
- Legumes: soybeans (tofu and other soy products), most beans.
- Grains: wheat, spelt, kamut. Buckwheat, amaranth
- Fruits: blackberries, raspberries, gooseberries, currants, kiwifruit, figs, and star fruit
- Vegetables: celery, beets, okra, sweet potatoes, rhubarb
- Other: cocoa, chocolate, and black tea.

When to use this diet: This diet it great to try if you have tried other ASD diets like GFCF and SCD and have reached a plateau and still have undesired symptoms. LOD is good to try for urinary problems and irritation, low energy and/or cognition, poor motor skills, GI or other pain within minutes or hours after eating, craving high oxalate food, continued constipation, diarrhea, or yeast overgrowth not relieved by other diets. Poor growth has been seen in children with high oxalates, and for these children LOD appears to correlate with growth spurts.

Pitfalls: LOD adds a further level of restriction to already restricted diets. Additionally, part of the problem may be due to vitamin K deficiency. It is theorized that by increasing vitamin K and adding other beneficial supplements, the low oxalate diet may not be necessary. However, this theory is new and may not address all concerns with oxalates. LOD limits vitamin C, an important nutrient for many children.

Clinical Experience: One of my clients had amazing results from this diet. Before LOD, he was on a modified version of GFCF, Body Ecology, and SCD. He was better on this diet, but always appeared to be battling yeast even after daily consumption of fermented foods, and immediately after every meal would rock and stim for at least 45 minutes. He also had a "mysterious rash" that would not go away. After being on the Low Oxalate Diet, his rocking and stimming disappeared along with the rash, and the yeast issue also improved greatly. The Low Oxalate Diet can be very effective, even when other diets have been tried.

See Appendix XIV for more information on the Low Oxalate Diet.

Feast without Yeast

This is one of the most basic and popular anti-candida diets. It is one of the least complicated candida diets. It is based on the book *Feast Without Yeast* by Bruce Semon. It reduces or eliminates the consumption of foods that feed candida: sugars, including fruit; fermented foods but not lactobacillus fermentations; moldy foods; and yeasts.

This diet can be used in conjunction with other diets. For the most part this diet has very sound, straight-forward principles. It is important to avoid sugars (cookies, sports bars, fruit juices, etc.) and greatly reduce or avoid refined carbohydrates such as pretzels, crackers, chips, and the like. Additionally moldy and aged foods including aged meats, cold cuts, and cheeses are prohibited. Also, avoiding baker's yeast found in bread is important.

The only discrepancy I have is with the fermented foods like live lacto-fermentations. Most "health programs" and yeast protocols will tell you to avoid fermented foods; however, lactobacillus-rich fermentations crowd out yeast. Especially helpful are lactobacillus fermentations like raw sauerkraut, kefir, and kombucha, which are highly beneficial at reestablishing the good bacteria and intestinal environment where yeast cannot survive. For this reason, I believe these kinds of fermented foods should be consumed liberally (see Fermented Foods in Part 3, Step #7, *Evolving the Diet: Nutrition Boosters*). Another beneficial fermented food, often eliminated on candida diets is raw, unpasteurized vinegars like apple cider vinegar, which is promoted on the Body Ecology yeast diet and can be very healthful. The only caveat to fermented foods is if someone has a strong IgG sensitivity to yeasts: in this case they need to proceed cautiously with the yeast-containing fermentations such as kombucha and kefir.

When to use this diet: It is a good place to start for someone with candida overgrowth. The principles of this diet are often applied to other diets. For example, a GFCF diet may also be low sugar and moldy foods. When adding probiotics creates regression from killing the yeast off and makes them impossible to do, the implementation of a candida diet such as this is very helpful first step. After the yeast is reduced from the diet, probiotics are often better tolerated and helpful.

Pitfalls: This diet is the easiest of the candida diets; however, sometimes further additions such as the Body Ecology principles of acid/alkaline and fermented foods are needed. Also, it is hard on anyone to do no sugar—especially children—so it can make this diet impossible for some.

Clinical Experience: I've seen this diet clear up inappropriate laughter and improve spaciness. It often is a diet that needs to be stuck to for six months. For those who cannot do no sugar, adding a small amount of fruit sugar is sometimes the best we can do with clients. While in some cases, this sugar makes the yeast very difficult to get rid of, usually with time, this low sugar diet in conjunction with more fermented foods and yeast killers works—albeit more slowly.

See Appendix IV for more information on a standard yeast diet.

Raw Food Diet

This diet has been used for years by a very small group of vegans called "raw foodists" to promote health. If you've heard of raw foodists, it may be through the growing number of famous raw foodists such as Woody Harrelson, Demi Moore (at one point), and chef Juliano Brotman. It is one of the newer diets in ASD circles, but the principles are not new and the concepts are sound. It uses the principles of enzymes and live, easily digestible foods. Raw foods are "hydrophilic colloidals," allowing them to draw liquids and digestive juices to enhance digestion. The enzymes, digestibility, and nutrient content of the foods increase dramatically with soaking and sprouting—a process used in raw food preparation. I definitely think there are sound principles that can be adopted from this diet.

I do not typically advocate this diet as a full raw food implementation, as it takes a certain digestive capacity to process some raw foods. Those with very compromised digestion have a difficult time with raw food. Although there are more enzymes in live, raw food, it is also true that certain foods like broccoli are more difficult to digest raw than in their cooked form. In fact raw foodists never eat cruciferous vegetables raw unless they have been otherwise processed. I usually combine the principles of raw foods and sprouting into other diets. The raw food diet does not need to be followed strictly so some aspects of it can be used in conjunction with any other diets.

When to use this diet: This diet is helpful to balance pH of the digestive tract, supporting the eradication of yeast and healing the gut. It is helpful for some people with digestive challenges and phenol issues. Some say that by implementing raw foods and balance pH they were able to eat more phenolic foods without reaction. The raw food diet has many principles that can be used in conjunction with other diets.

Pitfalls: While it sounds simple—eat food raw—there are many principles to understand to do this diet healthfully, as certain foods should not be eaten raw. This diet requires a varied diet with consumption of vegetables, beans, nuts, and is difficult for picky eaters. It is also quite time consuming and often requires days of forethought. Some people are most sensitive to uncooked food as cooking does breakdown certain necessary substances.

Clinical Experience: While it is helpful for digestion in some individuals and in theory, I find people with very compromised digestion have a difficult time digesting raw foods. One parent had particular success with using a raw food diet for her son. She felt that as he obtained a better acid/alkaline balance through the diet, he was able to process phenols better.

Paleolithic Diet

The Paleolithic diet (Paleo diet) is also known as the caveman diet or hunter-gatherer diet. It's high in fat and low in carbs, often considered one of many "low carb" diets. This diet is based on the premise that this is the diet humans evolved on for two million years during the Paleolithic period, only changing our diet "recently"—about 10,000 years ago when agriculture was invented. During this period cereal grains, starches, and legumes and dairy products were not consumed, and followers of this diet avoid plant foods that are not edible raw including grains, starchy vegetables (potatoes), beans, certain fruits and nuts, and refined sugars.

The diet focuses on meat, chicken, eggs, and fish. Ideally, the sources should be fresh; preferably grass-fed and organic beef, real free-range eggs from chickens who eat bugs and see the sun, and wild fish that eat what fish are meant to eat. Paleo also includes certain fruits, vegetables, nuts and seeds, leaves, berries, roots of plants, mushrooms, and honey.

The plant foods available in the diet are the same as those available in a raw food diet—the most digestible ones. However, the Paleo diet includes animal food as well and the food can be cooked.

When to use this diet: To me this is a stricter form of NT/WAP. It's similarly used for those needing a nourishing diet, but when grains and beans don't work regardless of soaking.

Pitfalls: If you don't eat animal food, this diet would be very difficult.

Clinical Experience: This diet is a little more simple SCD but more strict than NT/WAP. I usually use it as a modification when I want to expand SCD or restrict NT/WAP. Most of my clients choose SCD or NT/WAP over this diet but it seems to work similarly to these others improving digestion and nutrient reserves.

Gut and Psychology Syndrome (GAPS) Diet

This diet is essentially SCD, with particular emphasis on a few BED and NT/WAP principles of fermented foods and broths. See SCD for more information or *Gut and Psychology Syndrome* by Natasha Campbell-McBride for her specific suggestions on implementation and following the diet.

Ketogenic Diet

The ketogenic diet is a very strict diet specifically for seizures. Depending on the study, it has shown to be very effective, particularly for the high seizure (20 or more per day) children. I have not heard any one in the autism world using this diet. It is reserved for challenging seizure disorders where medications do not help.

The ketogenic diet is one of the few diets accepted by mainstream medicine. It was developed by the Mayo Clinic in the 1920's. This diet is 90 percent fat with the remaining ten percent divided between protein and carbohydrates. When this high of fat is consumed, the body goes into a state of ketosis, burning fat versus sugar for energy, and ketones build up. These ketones appear to prevent the electrical disturbances that cause seizures.

A large amount of this diet is butter, cream, peanut butter, cheese and similar high fat foods with small amounts of vegetables and fruit. Ironically, they do not seem to take toxic food additives into consideration as artificial sweeteners and colors are allowed, a recommendation I find fairly unbelievable since these artificial additives have been reported to trigger seizures in some people.

Butyrate converts to beta-hydroxybutyrate, a ketone produced during ketosis (during the ketogenic diet). According to a study discussed at the American Epilepsy Society 2004 Annual Meeting, "beta-hydroxybutyrate prevents hyperexcitability of neurons in rat brain slices exposed to acute oxidative stress, suggesting a neuroprotective effect" (Ben-Menachem, 2004). While I have not heard of anything definitive, it makes sense to reason that maybe one of the beneficial things about the ketogenic diet is the consumption of butter (high in butyrate). I wonder if adding butter to a monosaccharide diet (SCD) would provide some of the benefits without the overly strict ketogenic diet.

When to use it: The ketogenic diet is generally a last resort, after all other dietary options have been tried. As seizures can be caused by many toxins, try these other diets first: GFCF for food sensitivities, SCD or Body Ecology for dysboitic organisms and their toxic byproducts, and Feingold for phenols and artificial additives.

Pitfalls: This diet requires medical supervision and is very restrictive. It is not possible to meet all of your nutritional needs with the diet alone and requires a knowledgeable person to oversee the diet and recommend proper nutritional supplementation.

Clinical Experience: I have not worked with this diet. There are many stories of success for the ketogenic diet from those with severe seizures where nothing else had worked. However, there are reports of death from this diet as well.

Coping with Picky Eaters

Here's a note to parents—often frustrated parents—about children with picky eating habits. I address this issue throughout the book in greater detail, but it is worthwhile providing a summary of ideas here. There are many reasons for picky eating habits. My job (and your job as the parent or practitioner) is to try to understand why and work around this problem when possible. Picky eating can be due to:

1) Anxiety around trying anything new. This is common with ASD children and can be best addressed by going slowly and introducing a food many times without pressure to eat it. Ensure the rest of the dinner table is as stress free as possible.

2) Sensory issues around textures. Identify the texture desires and aversions of your child and then be creative. If a child likes only crispy, serve crispy raw vegetables or fry sweet potatoes or carrots chips. If a child only likes smooth texture, puree meat and use as a spread or inside a pancake recipe. Also look into sensory integration therapies and occupational therapy such as HANDLE, sound therapies, dry brushing, or have an occupational therapist work on oral defensiveness. (See note on sensory integration below.)

3) Food intolerances such as food sensitivities and phenols. If your child's diet is made up of high amounts of any one food, consider that this may be due to a food sensitivity. After removing these food addictions (gluten, casein, and apples), food choices often increase significantly.

4) Meat aversion. ASD kids can be affected by an inability to digest and process meat, sensory issues, or low muscle tone and a dislike for chewing. Look to improve nutrients, enzymes, and stomach acid (through HCl or bitter herbs). Also consider sensory integration therapy.

5) Food additives such as MSG and artificial ingredients. These chemicals can be addicting. MSG tricks the brain into thinking the food tastes good and the "excitability" can make other foods seem boring and tasteless. MSG and artificial colors and flavors can affect the neurotransmitters and become very addicting, creating a desire for only those foods.

It can take a long time to make changes—stick with it. Most of the time picky eating can be remedied or improved significantly. Here are a number of ideas to try with a picky eater to expand their food choices:

- Always provide food at the meal that your child likes in addition to the "new" food.
- Include a small portion of a new food and serve everyone at the table the same food.
- Involve your children in food preparation of the "new" food (i.e., ask them to count enough carrot sticks for everyone, serve the broccoli, or stir the fruit salad).
- A taste can be as small as 1/2 teaspoon. Let the child determine the amount he or she wants when you introduce a new food.
- Only offer one new food at a time. Let the child know whether it is sweet, salty, or sour. More than one food can be overwhelming.
- Children are more likely to try a new food if they have the option of not swallowing it. Show children how to carefully spit food into a napkin if they don't want to eat it.
- If at First You Don't Succeed, Try and Try Again! Research show that children may need to be offered a new food at least eight to ten times before they will try it. Use the Rule of 15, which says that you likely need to introduce a new food 15 times before a child accepts it.
- Try a new food in a texture you know your child prefers—crunchy, smooth, etc.
- Avoid being emotionally "attached" to your child expanding their diet because children sense your anxiety. Keep mealtime calm. Visualize your child eating/enjoying new healthy foods.
- Avoid forcing or pushing. It is very important to maintain trust.
- Choosing rewards or other encouragement can be helpful.
- Make sure the whole family participates. If Dad is a picky eater and isn't willing to eat the new foods, neither will the child.

A note on sensory integration: This can be a crucial piece of improvement. Eating restrictions are often related to sensory issues. For example, chewing crunchy foods is very loud for the person eating actually—notice for yourself some time. Also, texture issues with mushy foods are a big challenge. Low muscle tone can effect desire to chew meat. Because of this, there is limit to what a nutrition consultant can do. Explore sensory integration. There are a variety of auditory, visual, and somatic therapies for sensory sensitivity. HANDLE (www.handle.org) is one of these therapies. It addresses developmental milestones that may not have been reached for a variety of reasons. For example, crawling and sucking (specifically from the breast) create connections in the brain. If these milestones or developmental stages were not reached, sensory integration can be affected. This therapy involves home-based exercises you can do with your child in your own environment to simulate these developmental stages and connect these pathways. Explore sensory integration; there are many wonderful therapies and it is a worthwhile and often essential piece of the puzzle.

PART THREE

Holistic Guide to Nutrition Intervention

Holistic Nutrition Approach – Step by Step

The following is a diagram I created (Figure 6) on what "typically" provides the best path or approach to addressing the diet, nutrient, and biochemical issues involved with ASD. Of course, I put "typically" in quotation marks because as we have learned, each individual is unique with a different combination of genetics, environmental factors, and biochemical situations.

I created an order for things because, in general, it is often required that we address some issues before others. For example, we would need to clean up foods that are causing gut inflammation before healing the gut.

Additionally, the body is complex and certain systems are dependent on others. Sometimes we may need to go back and address an issue for a second time, after other factors have been addressed. When the circumstances are different, addressing the issue again often creates an additional level of improvement. An example of this is the gut, yeast, and mercury. While healing the gut is important before detox, it may be difficult to do so while mercury is present. In some respects it is beneficial to address the yeast first, for example, during detox. An existing condition of leaky gut (from yeast) allows the mercury to recirculate causing more damage, and certain high sulfur compounds used in chelation like DMSA and alpha lipoic acid feed yeast (adding to the gut problem). On the other hand, eliminating the yeast first may be difficult for several reasons. Yeast is often difficult to eradicate, and yeast often coexists with a state of mercury toxicity (possibly a protective mechanism or the yeast is feed on the mercury—we don't know this for sure yet.). The approach I've outlined functions best as a working guide, where you can change, repeat or skip steps as needed. Although we may start with certain things first, most interventions take years and most problems and solutions are interrelated.

I love Dr. Baker's "Tacks Law" to address the complexity of diet and supplementation—if you are sitting on a tack (food additives, gluten), no amount of aspirin (medication, vitamin C) will make it feel better; and if you are sitting on two tacks (two food sensitivities), the removal of one does not result in a 50% deduction in symptoms. The Tacks Law illustrates that when a condition is complex, much may need to be done before results can be seen sometimes. I think this is true, as no drug or supplement will "cure" the disorder and addressing half of the picture may not provide a significant improvement of symptoms. I suggest staying with it—further intervention is often required. I believe the reason these biochemical causes have been difficult to prove thus far is because they are complex and interdependent and scientific research uses the "one substance produces one result" model. As everyone is unique and these processes are interdependent, dramatic results are often not seen from a single intervention. Typically, what we see is that each intervention produces (a few large and) many small steps forward.

Figure 10B is a chart you can copy and put on your refrigerator to take notes, brainstorm, or chart progress for the *Holistic Nutrition Approach*, Figure 6.

Figure 6: Holistic Nutrition Approach – Step by Step

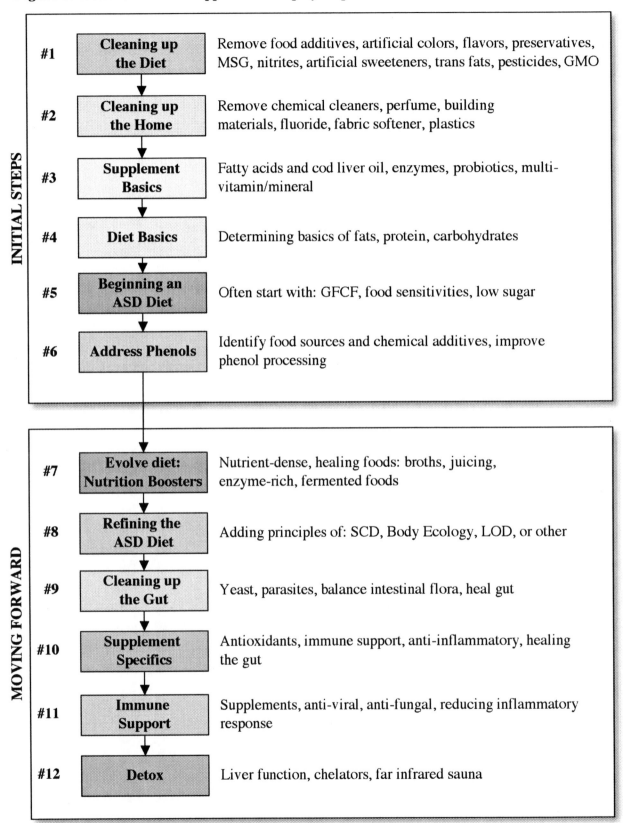

Holistic Nutrition Approach Notes and Observations

Step	Item	Notes and Observations
1	Cleaning up the Diet	
2	Cleaning up the Home	
3	Supplement Basics	
4	Diet Basics	
5	Beginning an ASD Diet	
6	Removing Food Intolerances	
7	Evolving the Diet: Nutrition Boosters	
8	Refining the ASD Diet	
9	Cleaning up the Gut	
10	Supplement Specifics	
11	Immune Support	
12	Detox	

#1 Cleaning up the Diet

So, where do you start? Most clinicians agree, the diet and gut offer the most impact and are the important places to start. This makes sense. If a child is creating a drug from artificial colors or opiates from dairy, in most cases, supplements will do little to address this. While enzymes and detoxifying agents can help with a toxic exposure, we would be chasing our tail continuously if we leave these substances in the diet.

Bryan Jepson, in his book *Changing the Course of Autism* says, "Diet changes often result in rapid improvements in both neurological and GI function, leading to better absorption of nutrients, decreased GI inflammation, and decreased immune system activation; subsequent improvement in sleep, bowel function, mood, and immunity follow."

Diet is integral to health, whether someone is on the spectrum or not, and many of the recommendations in this section can and should be applied to everyone in your family. The additives and ingredients I discuss here are unhealthy and often toxic to everyone. For some with ADHD, eliminating the following artificial ingredients is often enough to have a significant impact on and even complete elimination of symptoms. Start with these basics right away.

Sometimes when we first start a diet, "optimum nutrition" or nutrient-dense foods are not a priority, either for me or the parent. If they are not an initial objective, this is only short term. At first, I'm only worried about taking out the "toxic" foods. If there are addictions and food sensitivities, I'm more concerned about removing them 100% and substituting with (almost) anything. For example, if gluten is a problem, it is more important for me to remove gluten by adding a gluten-free waffle or treat in place of a piece of wheat bread. In this example, while I'm adding sugar through the substitution of (gluten-free) waffles with syrup for (gluten) toast—to the disgrace of nutritionists everywhere—my priority is to get the gluten out at any cost. The exception is that other toxic foods are never an acceptable substitution. If it is possible to substitute a healthy, low sugar, gluten-free replacement, then that, of course, would be ideal, but my priority at the beginning is removing the offending foods—pushing the nutrient dense foods may have to come later (and is discussed below).

Artificial Ingredients/Food Additives

The easiest things to get out of the diet—the ones with the most impact on behavior but least on taste—are the artificial ingredients. Synthetic food colorings and flavorings, in most cases, are made from petroleum products. Synthetic preservatives including BHA, BHT and TBHQ are also derived from petroleum. You wouldn't give your child a thimble full of motor oil! Would you? Since the end of World War II, Americans have been using preservatives with reckless abandon. For some reason, we think red maraschino cherries, that are redder than natural cherries and taste nothing like real cherries, are better than the real thing, and blue lollipops are normal. How can we make something taste more like strawberry than a strawberry itself? It can take some time for people to adjust to real flavor, and this process can be aided by some of the suggestions I made above regarding picky eaters; however, no one will miss artificial colors or preservatives.

As we discussed in the faulty sulfation section, artificial ingredients are very high in phenols—substances that require the sulfation detoxification pathway and PST to be working properly. As we know, in many people with autism and ADHD, these mechanisms are not working properly. For those individuals who have an inability to effectively metabolize phenolic amines, these substances are then toxic to the central nervous system and exacerbate autistic behavior. According to Feingold, these substances enter the brain and can cause disruption (Feingold, 2001). See Appendix XII for a list of phenolic additives to avoid.

How, then, does one remove these offending ingredients? Throw away foods you may have and refuse to buy any new ones which contain artificial ingredients: colors, preservatives, flavorings, BHA, BHT, annatto, emulsifiers, hydrolyzed vegetable protein, MSG, nitrates, nitrites, sorbates, sulfites. (Take the list you will find below with you when shopping, until you feel confident in reading labels on your own). Hot dogs are a favorite among many children; make sure they are nitrite-free, as these are carcinogenic (cancer-causing) compounds. Most natural food stores have substitutes for most of the foods with artificial ingredients. Try them. In most cases they are good. Often they even taste better and kids don't notice. In fact, remember, the artificial ingredients are typically used because they are covering up for inferior food quality and taste. Cereals and breads commonly contain BHA and BHT. Candy, cereals, chocolate, even some yogurt and fruit snacks, often contain artificial colors and flavors. While most artificial flavors will state something like "artificial strawberry flavor," it can be difficult sometimes to spot the artificials. Vanillin, for example, is artificial vanilla, but you will not find the word artificial. One must look carefully for "vanillin" as it is so similar to vanilla it can be missed. The good news is that for virtually every processed food, there is at least one choice of an additive-free version.

Regardless of what test results show, I would strongly urge you to remove these artificial flavors, colors, and preservatives from the entire family's diet. They are completely unnecessary, toxic to everyone (in varying degrees), and add further burden to already stressed livers.

MSG (Monosodium Glutamate)

MSG deserves special attention as we discuss what should be removed from the diet. In discussing MSG, we must also talk about neurological excitotoxins and neurological inflammation. MSG is an excitotoxin (a substance that can excite a brain cell to death). MSG creates a chemical message to the brain that these foods taste good, and a child can become very addicted and eventually self-select into a narrow range of only the foods that supply MSG. For example, when McDonald's chicken nuggets are the only nuggets eaten, you can bet it is the MSG making them taste "better."

MSG contains glutamate. Glutamate is an important excitatory neurotransmitter that is involved with both long and short term memory (maybe one reason for the amazing memories of some "savant autistics") and learning. Glutamate is converted to GABA, which in an inhibitory and calming neurotransmitter responsible for speech. Unfortunately, it is not as simple as more glutamate equals more GABA. If you have too much glutamate in the diet, the conversion to GABA is inhibited. Furthermore, when there is too much glutamate that can not be processed (as is what happens with many ASD kids who consume MSG) the glutamate becomes toxic to neurons, creating neurological inflammation and neuron death. Neurological inflammation is discussed extensively by Dr. Amy Yasko as an important factor in autistic spectrum disorders (more at http://www.ch3nutrigenomics.com/phpBB2/welcome.html).

Additionally MSG consumption can cause headaches, migraines, hyperactivity, excess acid and heartburn, diarrhea, nausea, bloating, depression, respiratory problems, and more.

Read labels very carefully, MSG can be disguised or hidden as:
- MSG, monosodium glutamate, and glutamic acid (found in some amino acid blends)
- Gelatin
- Yeast extract, autolyzed yeast
- Hydrolyzed soy protein, hydrolyzed corn protein, or any hydrolyzed protein
- Hydrolyzed corn gluten
- Calcium caseinate, sodium caseinate
- Textured protein
- Monopotassium glutamate
- "Natural Flavors"
- Surprisingly, even processed foods sold at natural foods stores often contain hidden MSG.

Soups, broths, gravies, imitation meat products, and many meat and cheese flavored foods often contain MSG. Be careful of most protein powders, they are often hydrolyzed protein.

Interestingly, gluten and casein also contain high levels of glutamate and aspartate (another excitotoxin described next). This is likely an additional reason for prevalent gluten and casein intolerances.

Artificial Sweeteners

Eliminate all artificial sweeteners: NutraSweet, Equal, aspartame, Sweet 'N Low, saccharine, sucralose/Splenda. Artificial sweeteners cause further sugar cravings, deplete nutrients from the body including chromium which helps metabolize sugars, and many have been implicated in causing cancer. Aspartate is found in aspartame (or NutraSweet). Aspartate is an excitotoxin (like glutamate) and hence most of what applies to neurotoxicity with MSG applies to asparatame. Splenda has a wonderful marketing campaign that it is "made from sugar." It is chemically derived from sugar. In a five step patented process, three chlorine molecules are added to a sucrose molecule, and as it does not occur in nature, the body can not process it well and certainly cannot utilize it the same as a natural sugar. There has been a history of approval and use of artificial sweeteners, many of which have later been implicated in causing negative health effects, including cancer.

If yeast is present and no sugars are tolerated, use stevia or xylitol (two natural sweeteners). Stevia is derived from the stevia plant and while sweet does not raise blood sugar or feed yeast. Xylitol, also known as birch sugar, is a natural sweetener that does not raise blood sugar or feed yeast. However, be sure you don't assume all xylitol comes from birch bark; more and more it is derived from corn—a common food sensitivity. Glycerin can be used if someone is on SCD and can't do honey because of phenols.

Trans Fats and Hydrogenated Fats

Eliminate all trans fatty acids (or trans fats as they are commonly known) and all hydrogenated fats. These fats do not occur in nature. They are created in a lab using high heat and heavy metals to turn vegetable oils that are liquid at room temperature into solids. Chemically, they resemble plastic more closely than they do food. Therefore, they are not broken down and processed well by the body. As mentioned earlier, trans fats fill the omega fatty acid receptors, causing even more problems for ASD kids who are generally low in omega-3 fatty acids.

Trans fats include: hydrogenated oil, partially hydrogenated oil, margarine, industrial deep fried foods, commercial peanut butter (Skippy and Jif types of peanut butter as opposed to the natural peanut butters), and commercial mayonnaise (unless specified non-hydrogenated).

Pesticides

Pesticides are designed to kill. While they quickly kill small organisms, they slowly "kill" larger organisms such as humans, and especially children. These substances kill cells, disrupt cellular function, add a toxic load to the body, and must be processed by the detoxification system. Single pesticides are tested for short trials on grown adult males. When companies test for "safety," they never test on children, never test for their long-term effects, and never test for their synergistic impact. More impartial studies have shown that the synergy between several pesticides is much more toxic than single pesticides (just as we learned about toxic metals), and in agriculture several if not dozens of different insecticides, fungicides, herbicides, and bactericides are used.

Avoid pesticides in produce, dairy and meat. Conventional meat and dairy also contain hormones, antibiotics, and other additives. Eat only organic whenever possible.

Genetically Modified Organisms (GMOs)

GMOs are "foods" (I call them foods loosely) where scientists change the DNA of the living organism. This is not simple hybridization like crossing a pear with an apple and getting an asian pear. GMOs contain DNA from viruses, bacteria, other foods (that people may be allergic to), or any other DNA fragments. The marketing campaigns for these companies tout that we will be able to grow more food for the world by creating disease and pest resistant plants, and participate in other humanitarian efforts. However, the reality is that GMO crops can have smaller yields than non-GMO crops, not larger. Additionally, the genetically modified plants are created to endure the spraying of their company's pesticides, such as Monsanto's herbicide, Round Up. The seeds have a "suicide gene" so they can not reproduce. The biotech companies do not allow for the saving and reuse of seed from season to season and require farmers to buy the seed from them each year (www.organicconsumers.org). They sell the plant seeds and chemical herbicides to the farmers—creating more profit for the biotech companies and more enslavement for the farmers.

In her paper, *The Health Hazards of Genetically Engineering Foods*, Laurie Lynch, ND, PhD candidate-Nutrition, compiled research revealing that some varieties of GMO foods have been shown to have significant differences in fat and carbohydrate content. Anywhere from 12% to 20% drop in protein, certain vitamins, and phytochemicals as compared to non-GM varieties (Lynch). Dr. Lynch cites the following facts:

- "GM maize show significant differences in fat and carbohydrate content, compared with non-GM maize."
- In another study of GM Vica Faba, a bean in the same family as soy, there was also an increase in estrogen levels, which raises health issues—especially in infant soy formulas
- Some GE potatoes showed a 20% drop in protein quality, lower disease-fighting capabilities, and nutrition.
- A variety of GM tomato had about 15% less vitamin C.
- "According to Monsanto's own tests, Roundup Ready soybeans contain 29'% less of the brain nutrient choline, and 27% more trypsin inhibitor (a potential allergen that interferes with protein digestion), …lower levels of phenylalanine, an essential amino acid that affects levels of phytoestrogens. And levels of lectins, …allergens, are nearly double in the transgenic variety."
- "…cows ingesting GE soybeans have exhibited higher levels of fat in their milk."
- "Roundup Ready soybeans showed as much as a 20% drop…" in certain phytochemicals."
- The use of rBGH also contributes to "increased antibiotic residues in the milk, resulting from higher rates of udder infections…"
- "Milk from cows injected with rBGH contains higher levels of pus, bacteria, and fat."

Further information about GMO foods:
- They do not need to be labeled.
- People have died from undisclosed allergies to the protein from brazil nuts (Cummins:2000) and other unknown compounds.
- There are no long-term safety studies.
- They contaminate organic crop with cross-pollination from nearby farms, rendering the organic plants no longer organic and unable to be sold overseas or as organic.

Eat organically! The main GMO crops are corn, soy, canola, and cottonseed. For these foods, always get organic unless it's GMO-free. To be organic, no GMOs can be present.

Consider writing to you government representative. We should have labeling for GMOs. We have the right to know what we are eating. And if the biotech companies really believe there is nothing wrong with their food, they should be happy to label it.

Step one, *Cleaning up the Diet*, makes one of the biggest impacts and is easy to do once you get the hang of it. It will make a noticeable difference in the health of your whole family. The key is to read labels, specifically the list of ingredients, not just the marketing fluff on the package. Photocopy the following chart and keep it with you in your handbag or on the refrigerator to use as a reference until identifying these toxins becomes second nature.

FOOD

AVOID	BETTER CHOICES
• Table salt with aluminum • Baking powder with aluminum • Artificial colors • Artificial flavors and vanillin • Preservatives • Nitrates/nitrites • MSG: Monosodium glutamate, hydrolyzed vegetable/soy protein, hydrolyzed corn protein, autolyzed yeast, yeast extract/food, caseinate • Trans fats • Pesticides • GMO foods • Farm-raised fish with PCBs • Time-released pharmaceutical drugs • Mercury in fish • Aluminum cans (often lined with plastic) • Antacids with aluminum • Fluoride tablets • Artificial sweeteners and fats • Non-organic poultry and rice (may contain arsenic)	• Eat organic, locally grown produce. • Avoid produce grown in other countries where guideline are less strict • When non-organic, peel and wash produce (Dr. Bronner's and special produce washes work well) • Read labels. • Buy foods free of artificial colors, flavors and preservatives. There are additive-free versions of virtually every food. • Buy salt and baking powder free of aluminum

Resources: Identifying safe and artificial ingredients in food

www.feingold.org

#2 Cleaning up the Home

Cleaning up your household environment is just as important as cleaning up the diet. Household toxins are bad for the whole family and have a significant negative impact. These changes are also easy to implement and therefore a reasonable and important second step.

As detoxification is often impaired for those with ASD, cleaning up chemicals in the environment is key. This does not just include obvious items like insecticides but basic cleaning supplies and body care products. Think of the liver as a funnel: it can only handle so many toxins at one time. There are many things we do not have control over that the liver must process: (1) those things made inside the body (endogenous) such as used hormones and the byproducts of both good and bad microorganisms, and (2) those things from outside the body (exogenous) such as the air we breathe and the pesticides at the park. Because we live in a world with many toxins, reducing exposure where we can is important. Many of these toxin household substances, besides being poisons, also cause cancer and disease. Many of them are also phenolic and therefore need to be processed by the sulfation pathway. Add to that the fact that the vast majority are bad for our environment, and you can see why removing these from your household forever is an excellent idea

Chlorine Bleach and other Chemical Cleaners

The process of creating chlorine bleach gives off dioxin, one of the most toxic substances on earth. The fumes are toxic, so avoid using chlorine bleach in your home or in laundry. Chlorine inhibits the stomach's ability to produce hydrochloric acid (HCl), which diminishes digestion, and also acts as a "disinfectant," killing the good bacteria in the gut. Chlorine destroys unsaturated essential fatty acids like omega-3s and 6s. Avoid paper products bleached with chlorine. Avoid chlorine in swimming pools and tap water when possible. Since swimming provides so many benefits, instead of avoiding swimming, try avoiding the chlorine. For your own pool, consider an ionizer to disinfect instead of chlorine. Pool ionizers cuts down on 70-80% of the chlorine needed; however, they use copper and silver to disinfect so for individuals with copper excess or extreme zinc deficiency, this also may have its set of challenges. More and more pools in hotels and resorts are switching to salt water pools. Parents often report positive results when using Epsom salt baths or creams before and after their child goes into a swimming pool. To avoid chlorine in tap water, get a filter for the tap and shower, or a whole house filter.

Perfumes or Fragrance

Avoid all artificial fragrances. Artificial fragrances contain dozens of chemicals including xylene, toluene, phthalates, and other chemicals that are toxic to the brain and liver, and cause cancer. They must be processed by the sulfation pathway and they add a large burden to the liver. This means mom and dad must avoid perfume and cologne. If your child spends time with another caregiver, be sure to ask that person to follow these same suggestions. Natural essential oils can by used as perfume and in body care products when tolerated by the child.

Building Materials and Solvents (paint, aerosols)

Building materials include carpets, fabrics, foam padding, paints, lacquers, etc. All of these off-gas volatile organic compounds (VOCs). According to the EPA's website, the health effects of VOCs include, "Eye, nose, and throat irritation; headaches, loss of coordination, nausea; damage to liver, kidney, and central nervous system. Some [volatile] organics can cause cancer in animals; some are suspected or known to cause cancer in humans." Some of these building materials contain heavy metals and other toxins. Additionally, in new cars, the "new car smell" is the result of the film on the inside of the windshield and other materials off-gassing VOCs.

These substances are endocrine disrupters and neurotoxins. They are very difficult to detoxify, especially in an overburdened system. Use healthier, environmentally friendly paints and building materials whenever possible. When you need to paint, look for low VOC (Volatile Organic Compounds) paints with less than 100 gm/l.

Additionally, many of these building materials (as well as mattresses and infant sleepwear) contain flame retardant with many harmful industrial chemicals including the heavy metal antimony. See the *Resources* section for safe non-toxic products.

Fluoride

Fluoride is a highly toxic substance. A great book written on this subject is *The Slow Poisoning of America*, where the authors, John and Michelle Erb, describe their own son's poisoning with fluoride. On my website (www.healthfulliving.org) there is a link to a report by the Greater Boston Physicians for Social Responsibility on the toxic effects of fluoride. In this paper they reference scientific studies done on fluoride and its effects on brain development, childhood IQ, and hyperactivity. Fluoride also inhibits the stomach's ability to produce HCl. Allergy and skin irritation are known side effects of fluoride. Even death can result from excess fluoride especially in children (as they are smaller than adults and tend to swallow fluoride treatments).

Contrary to popular opinion among dentists, there are no conclusive studies that fluoride is beneficial for strong teeth. In fact, excess fluoride causes brittle teeth and bones. Populations that fluoridate water have no difference in the number of dental cavities than those that don't. Why do we believe fluoride is good for us, and why have we not heard otherwise? If I can be so bold, this is the same industry that STILL tells us that putting mercury in your teeth is safe.

Frequently I see children with autism with prescriptions for fluoride tablets when the local water is not fluoridated. Parents should do their own research, decide what they feel comfortable with, and speak with their physician and health care team.

Fabric Softeners

Fabric softeners contain toxic artificial fragrance and chemicals to bind the fragrance. These chemicals are proven neurotoxins—that is, they kill nerve and brain cells. The fabric softener chemicals coat the clothing (it's difficult to even wash out) and are in contact with the individual's skin all day and all night, even on the pillowcase they sleep on. Fabric softeners should be avoided entirely by the whole family. Companies such as Seventh Generation make liquid fabric softeners free of artificial fragrance and the toxic chemicals present in commercial fabric softeners, or better yet, skip them all together.

Petroleum Jelly and Mineral Oil

Petroleum jelly, Vaseline, Chapstick, and Johnson's baby oil are all made from petroleum products. These are high in phenols and because they absorb through the skin, they must be processed by the liver and the sulfation pathway. Use Unpetroleum Jelly and petroleum free lip balms and body oils.

Plastics/Phthalates

Plastics are toxic. They stay in the body for many decades and disrupt hormonal and neurotransmitter balance. They overburden the detoxification system and are basically "hardened petroleum"—especially difficult on those with phenol and sulfation challenges. While there is no "best" plastic, there is a "worst" plastic—polyvinylchloride (PVC). Phthalates are chemicals used to soften PVC, causing the chemicals to leak into the food or from the toy more easily. Phthalates have shown damage to the liver, the kidneys, and the lungs. Phthalates are plasticizers or soft plastics that are used to make things sticky, stretchy, and durable. Plastics and phthalates are used in hairspray, synthetic fragrance, nail polish, teethers, toys, new cars, and many more products. Commercial cling wraps, bottles, teethers and soft squeeze toys for young children, beach balls, bath toys, dolls, and lunchboxes are made with PVC.

We once thought that while these soft plastics were harmful, hard plastic like those used in Nalgene bottles and the 5-gallon water bottles were safe. However, now we know Bisphenol-A (BPA) found in these hard plastics is very dangerous. Being one of many known endocrine disruptors, BPA causes miscarriages and affects development, intelligence, memory, learning, and behavior. BPA and phthalates have been shown to have a significant effect on prostate size, epididymal weight, penis size, and anogenital distance in newborn boys (Gupta, 2000).

Despite what you have heard, plastics do leach into whatever they come in contact with. Don't store food or carry water in plastic. Especially do not let food or liquids get hot in plastic. For example, do not pour hot leftovers into plastic storage containers, do not leave water bottles in the car, and do not microwave in plastic.

Cooking

Cast iron and enameled cast iron are good options for cookware. Stainless steel pots and pans are also good options; however, stainless steel can contain high levels of nickel. Buy stainless steel that attracts a magnet—these are much lower in nickel. If you can find the old VisionWare by Corning Ware, they are also great to cook with. Do not use aluminum (where the cooking surface is aluminum), Teflon-coated, or copper. Especially, do not use Teflon. I know they are easy and non-stick but there have been many studies showing how toxic this material is. Even if they are new and unscratched I would not use them.

I highly recommend not using a microwave. Microwaving denatures the protein (ever seen a microwaved egg?) and depletes the nutrient content significantly. If you need to start with other suggestions first because this is too overwhelming, start slowly. Begin to heat food in a pot or pan on the stove, the oven, or a toaster oven. You will quickly begin to see that you really don't need and won't miss the microwave.

Store food in freezer-safe mason jars, glass or Pyrex storage containers. If the lid is plastic that's fine as long as the food will not touch it. Many people wrap food in parchment paper before wrapping it in something like aluminum foil for long term freezer storage.

PERSONAL CARE

AVOID	BETTER CHOICES
• Deodorant with aluminum • Synthetic fragrances • Nail polish • Hairspray, hair gels, mousses with phthalates • Soaps with parabens • Makeup with phthalates, lead, synthetic ingredients • Shampoos • Lice-killing products • Infant sleepwear with flame-retardant (antimony) • Toothpaste with fluoride and artificial ingredients • Sunscreen (chemical-based) • Bleached paper products especially tampons • Amalgam fillings	• Choose make up, nail polish, and other body care products that are free of phthalates. • Use tampons and other paper products free of chlorine bleach • Buy non-aluminum deodorant • Use safe dental materials. Avoid amalgam fillings and plastic resins. • Use a chemical free sunscreen. Spend more time in the shade and avoid large amounts of sunscreen. • See resource list and chose body care products free of phthalates, strong detergents and synthetic ingredients.

Toxic and non-toxic cosmetics and body care products
www.nottoopretty.org

www.cosmeticsdatabase.com/

HOME

AVOID	BETTER CHOICES
• Plastic toys • Vinyl and PVC toys and lunchboxes (also contain lead) • Teethers with phthalates • Candles with lead wicks • Paints with VOCs • Paint thinners • Adhesives • Fabric softener • Cigarette smoke • Styrofoam • Microwave ovens • Plastic water bottles, food storage containers, baby bottles • Teflon pans • Aluminum pans • Detergents and chemical cleaners • Antibacterial soaps • Chlorine bleach • Water with chlorine, chloramine, fluoride or lead • Lead in dishware, pipes, or paint • Carpeting • Wood products (plywood, chipboard) • Mildew and mold in home • Pesticide spraying • Arsenic-treated wood in playgrounds or decks (green-tinted) • New cars (dashboard, upholstery) • EMF (electro-magnetic frequencies) • Dry cleaning	• Store food in glass. Do not store food in plastic wrap. • Look for PVC free film wrap. Some cellophane wraps are naturally made from cellulose. • Buy toys and teethers without phthalates. See resource list of websites. • Use glass or a stainless steel water bottle • Reduce your use of plastic and look for non-chlorinated plastics with the 2,4, or 5 "recycling number" • Use natural cleaners • Best to buy a reverse osmosis, carbon, ionic or other water filter. • Install a "point of entry" water filter (clean water throughout house including bathing) if possible • Get a shower filter that takes out chlorine • Purchase an air filter or dehumidifier (for mildewy environments) • If you have your own pool, use an ozone or other safer pool disinfectant • Purchase safe decorating, construction and building materials • Go to environmentally-friendly dry cleaner • Use natural herbal or biodynamic insect repellents around the home

Resources: Products for a safe home and healthy child

www.checnet.org - Children's' Health Environmental Coalition

www.greenhome.com - Great resource for natural apparel, toys, bedding

www.ahappyplanet.com - "Organic fibers for everyday and every night

#3 Supplement Basics

Adding some basic supplements is a good thing to do while you are trying to figure out what and how to feed your child. A few of the supplements that seem to offer the best results with the fewest problems are enzymes, probiotics, and cod liver oil. Enzymes and probiotics have very little flavor and are fairly easy to add. Cod liver oil (CLO) may be a bit more difficult but good flavored ones are available. The difficult part with CLO (in addition to the smell) is that an oil feels funny from a sensory perspective to swallow by itself. Mix it in a small amount juice or better yet, a smoothie where it can be more suspended. However, make it a small "shot glass" size as the fish oil will flavor it a bit and it's easier to chug a small amount down.

While a good quality multivitamin/mineral formula can provide a wide range of nutrients the child may need, they are not always the best place to start. Multis have so many nutrients that reactions are common in sensitive children, and the flavor is often strong due to the B-vitamins. For this reason it is often preferred to start with some individual nutrients until you determine what a child does well with and whether a multi is tolerated.

Some of the basic supplements to consider first are in the left column. There are additional supplements in the right column that I typically add after the first list. However, as everyone is different, you can begin to implement any of these that seem most helpful. See the list of benefits and common uses in *Impact of Nutrients* to help you determine which you might want to try first.

Basic supplements	Second level supplements
Enzymes	B6
Probiotics	Vitamin E
Cod liver oil	Folic acid/folinic/5MTHF
Zinc	B12
Magnesium	Selenium
Calcium	GLA
Vitamin C	Multivitamin/mineral formula

Always start slowly with any supplement, at a fraction of the standard dose, and work up to the standard dose. Also only add one supplement at a time to identify potential reactions. Document responses from supplements by keeping a record of when you add them and any positive or negative reactions you see. This will help to determine if they are helpful or whether you need to try something else. See diet record samples in *Progress and Regression*.

Healing the gut is essential. If the gut is not healed enough to absorb the nutrients, the nutrients are not as effective as they could be. Enzymes and probiotics will help to do this, so a good time to add them in is at the beginning. As the gut heals, the vitamins and minerals will absorb better. Be aware, though, that healing the gut completely can take years and for many children, healing the gut is impossible without supplementation. This is why they are simultaneous goals.

#4 Diet Basics

Now that we have cleaned the toxins and toxic foods out of the diet, let's discuss what *to* eat. As autistic children are often very picky eaters and set on routine, diet is not an easy area to change. I have clients who will only eat certain textures. Also, as discussed earlier, sensory sensitivities are a common reason for many self-imposed food restrictions. I have also seen and heard of food restrictions clearing up when yeast or viral issues are addressed. Several clients will only eat food of pureed or liquid texture. The parents have observed or believe this to be a sensory issue—either to texture or to sound (notice how loud crunchy foods are when you chew them). One very helpful thing is to try to mimic the child's current food choices, textures, and flavors as much as possible to make the conversion easier. We have found that some kids will eat vegetables or *anything* if it is in their preferred form. For the situation with blended foods, some kids will eat rice milk, cooked grain, green vegetables, and chicken blended…together. Be creative.

The previous discussions on substances that need to be taken out of the diet are "mandatory" changes. The following suggestions are "ideal" suggestions to aim for over time. Protein (vegetable sources, and "clean" or organic meats), complex carbohydrates (fruits, vegetables, whole grains, beans and legumes, root vegetables), and good fats (flax, nuts/seeds, avocado, olive oil) are the areas to focus on. Focus on organic produce and meat, whole and unprocessed foods, fruits and vegetables, and as much variety as possible. When in doubt focus on eating a "traditional diet"—think of what people ate for hundreds or thousands of years, before modern processing of foods came about, and look into the Nourishing Traditions/Weston A. Price diet.

Be patient and build trust with the child. Adding new foods to the diet might take months and the transition is an ongoing process. With that said, give your child the benefit of the doubt. I've seen many children who have adapted quite well to new dietary choices, even to the surprise of the parent who thought the picky eating habits were going to cause a big problem. While you can be stern and "force" what they cannot eat, you cannot "force" them to EAT any food. If you are going to be firm, be firm on taking out toxic foods. When you are introducing new foods, go slowly, be patient, build trust. Do not force it: you will lose. It may take you months but eventually you will get there.

One child I worked with would not touch meat but three days after being gluten- and casein-free, he started eating several different types of meat cooked in a variety of ways. Another child, a girl I worked with, did not eat any vegetables and within a month after being GFCF she began eating vegetables for the first time. I have heard story after story of this happening, and it makes sense. If you have access to your food addiction, why branch out and try anything else, as nothing can compare to the high you get from eating your "fix." However, once the cravings subside and the addictive chemicals are out of the system, new choices open up.

Let's start with some of the basics. Below is a chart of calories and grams of protein, as well as a percentage breakdown of macronutrients (protein, fat, carbs) in the average child's diet based on age. These are just a guideline. Of course, based on digestive healthy and biochemistry, individual amounts and percentages will vary.

I don't expect my clients to count calories or grams on a regular basis, but it can be helpful to do a diet analysis if you have a child with a very restrictive diet. I want to stress that this chart is more of a rough guideline. You will see that the ranges are very broad. I would not restrict calories to try to fit into this model. It is more for children with very poor eating habits so that parents can get an idea of the minimum protein and calories that are important for many children.

	2-4 years	4-6 years	6-11 years	12-15 years
Calories	1300-1600	1600-2100	2100-2800	Girls 2000-2300 Boys 2600-3000
Protein	23-60 gr	30-80 gr	35-95 gr	45-85 gr 45-95 gr

Protein   7-20% of total calories
Fat: 25-45% + of total calories
Carbohydrates: 40-60%+ of total calories

Be aware that there are many exceptions to this chart. For example, children with high ammonia will need much less protein. Children with leaky guts may need higher levels of calories. Children with gallbladder or fat digestion problems may need to reduce fat. There are further nuances of diet to determine which end of the range a child would want to be on throughout this section.

Fat

Fat is my favorite subject. It is the macronutrient about which the most misinformation has been spread in the mainstream and nutrition world. A low fat diet is always touted as superior. However, fat is absolutely crucial for many things including brain development, hormone balance, formation of the cell membrane, skin health, creation of energy, reduction (or increase) in inflammation, absorption of nutrients. The list is very long.

Don't be afraid of fat. I typically recommend that fat is at least 30% of the diet, and many children do well with 40% or more. Breast milk is 53% fat (25% saturated). However, proceed slowly as not everyone can digest fats well, including many with autism. High fat may be problematic for those with high oxalates, gallbladder/bile imbalances, and enzyme insufficiency (lipase enzyme helps). Signs of poor fat digestion include stool that is light tan or gray in color and/or large in volume. Sometimes stool will float when there is maldigestion but not always. Flatulence can be malodorous, but this is also a sign of yeast or dysbiosis. A Comprehensive Digestive Stool Analysis (CDSA) can test fat absorption. (see *Assessments* in the *Impact of Nutrients* section).

For someone who needs increased bile production for digestion of fats, taurine can be helpful as it is an ingredient in bile salts. Bile salts are also sold as supplements in liver/gallbladder formulas and can also be taken directly. Lipase aids fat digestion as well.

It's important to make sure fats are not oxidized in the body. Children with autism are often limited in antioxidants and have a lot of oxidative stress. Fatty acid balance and oxidation can be tested with a fatty acid profile (see *Assessments* in the *Impact of Nutrients* section). Supplementing with vitamin E can help prevent oxidation of fats.

There are many types of fats and it's important to have well-rounded consumption. The fats include:

Omega-3	Omega-6	Omega-9	Saturated Fat
Fish oil or cod liver oil	Borage oil (GLA) Evening primrose oil (GLA) Black currant oil (GLA)	Olive oil	Coconut oil
Flax seed oil	Nuts/seeds and their oil Hemp seeds/oil (GLA)	Avocado	Palm/Red Palm oil
DHA and EPA supplements	Grapeseed oil	Nuts/seeds	Animal fats such as ghee/dairy, bacon
	AVOID Vegetable oil: canola, safflower, corn, soy.		

Omega-3 is one of the most important oils for everyone but especially babies and children. Omega-3 has two important components, EPA and DHA. EPA is required for brain function and DHA is essential for brain development. . It is crucial for proper neurological function. Bock states that, "DHA contributes to the function of the brain cell receptors, which allow the entry of important neurological chemicals, including neurotransmitters and hormones" (Bock 2007). Omega-3 comes from two main sources: cold water fish and flax seeds. I don't recommend fish for children with autism because of the mercury content and their poor detoxification capability. Fish oil is a better option for omega-3 as the toxins can be filtered out. Flax seeds can be helpful for constipation. While flax seeds and flax oil have omega-3, the body needs to convert the alpha-linolenic acid (ALA) into EPA and DHA through an enzyme, delta 6 desaturase, which requires certain nutrients (B6, magnesium, zinc) and freedom from certain conditions (high insulin, toxins, alcohol). For these reasons, and because cod liver oil (CLO) has the additional benefit of vitamins A and D, I prefer fish oil and cod liver oil.

You can get too much omega-3, so don't go overboard. Keep fatty acids in balance by dosing based on information identified in fatty acid test results, according to the label, or your practitioner (see the Impact of Nutrients section for more information on fatty acid testing and fish oil).

Omega-6: Omega-6 is also important. We need a 4:1 ratio of omega-6 to omega-3. That is, we need four times as much omega-6 as omega-3; however, most Americans get twenty times the omega-6 compared to omega-3. This creates a fatty acid imbalance. Most of us don't need to supplement omega-6 with the exception of possibly GLA. Children who don't seem to tolerate omega-3 in the form of cod liver oil may in fact be deficient in omega-6 and may require omega-6 supplementation. Fatty acid imbalances and even deficiencies can be difficult to determine without testing. A fatty acid profile can give you information that may prove helpful for supplementation (see the Impact of Nutrients section for more information on fatty acid testing).

Linoleic acid is a common type of omega-6, often elevated in children with ASD. Too much linoleic acid will decrease IgA, which is an important part of the immune response in the gut and is needed to protect the intestines. Oils that contain a high proportion of linoleic fatty acids are safflower, corn, soy, canola, and nut oils. Avoid these. They are often oxidized and imbalance the other fatty acids.

Omega-9: We don't hear too much about Omega-9. Olive oil and avocado are the most common form of omega-9. We can make omega-9 so it's not essential and most people don't need to supplement with more – but getting some in the diet is good.

Saturated Fat: My biggest pet peeve is when people lump saturated fats together with trans fats. They only have one thing in common—they are both solid at room temperature. Period. That is where the similarities end. Trans fat, as we discussed in step #1 "Cleaning up the Diet," are toxic fats that imbalance the good fats and cause many health problems. Saturated fat does not go rancid and is a good oil to cook with at higher heat (as is the omega-6 oil grapeseed oil).

Saturated fat is very important and healthful in the right proportions and in the right quality. Saturated fat is important for:
- Cell Membranes – should be 50% saturated fatty acids.
- Brain – development of the brain in babies and children.
- Bones – saturated fats help the body put calcium in the bones.
- Liver – saturated fats protect the liver from alcohol and other poisons.
- Lungs – can't function without saturated fats—protects against asthma.
- Kidneys – can't function without saturated fats.
- Immune System – enhanced by saturated fats—fights infection.
- Essential Fatty Acids – work together with saturated fats.

Saturated fat comes from both plant and animal sources. Of course, as only animals make cholesterol, plant oils, such as coconut, do not contain cholesterol. One of my favorite saturated fats is **coconut oil**. Coconut oil contains many antifungal and antiviral components. It is high in caprylic acid, which helps kill yeast. Coconut oil also contains high amounts of lauric acid, a potent anti-microbial and one of the abundant fatty acids in breast milk. Coconut oil has anti-inflammatory effects. Coconut oil will also enhance thyroid function and can aid weight loss for those who are overweight. Coconut oil enhances the absorption of minerals. Coconut oil is one of the few medium chain triglycerides (MCT) in the diet, and the medium chain fatty acids do not require energy for absorption and do not require bile salts making them more easily digested and absorbed. They are used immediately to create energy.

When purchasing a coconut oil to eat raw, look for an extra virgin or virgin, since this oil is unrefined and still has the nutrients, enzymes, and beneficial fatty acids intact. For frying and high heat cooking, the expresser-pressed coconut oil is an economical choice. Because it is processed (but without chemicals) it does not have the same level of nutrient as virgin; however as heat destroys some nutrients anyway it is a reasonable choice for high heat cooking. I like Wilderness Family Farms (they even have coconut milk in glass) and Tropical Traditions.

Cholesterol: While animal fats contain cholesterol, this is not a negative thing. Cholesterol is essential for many functions. In fact, all hormones are built from a cholesterol molecule. Additionally, cholesterol aids brain function, boosts mental performance, aids digestion, builds strong bones, and serves many more integral body functions. In spite of what we've been told, cholesterol is not the *cause* of heart disease nor is it necessarily a marker for problems. Trans fats, high sugar, high homocysteine, high c-reactive protein (a marker of inflammation), are far more concerning for heart disease than cholesterol. For detailed information on the myths regarding cholesterol, I would highly recommend *The Cholesterol Myths* by Uffe Ravnskov, M.D., PhD. For now, know cholesterol that is essential for children and as long as you are getting good sources of animal fat, it is healthy when in balance with other fats.

Protein

Adequate protein is important in order to obtain the building blocks—that is, essential amino acids—for muscle and tissue growth and repair. Furthermore, protein intake is essential for neurotransmitter function, immune response, hormone function, enzyme function, and detoxification. Because of bio-individuality amounts required may vary. Some children cannot process protein well. People with high ammonia, low HCl, low zinc, low B6, or low iron may have difficulties processing protein. In protein metabolism (using protein for energy) the waste product nitrogen needs to be converted in the urea cycle into urea and excreted in the urine—otherwise, ammonia will build up. High ammonia can be due to too high protein intake when there is a problem in the urea cycle or dysbiotic bugs in the gut (creating more ammonia). For certain children (Yasko has identified a polymorphism with CBS, cystathionine beta synthase), both animal and plant protein intake needs to be reduced fairly significantly for a period of time. Yasko uses yucca to reduce ammonia levels, although yucca is high in oxalates. See more on reducing ammonia in the *Seizures* section.

Earlier in this section I provided some ranges for protein. The range is wide is it varies greatly from person to person. If your child eats meat or eggs a couple times a day, they probably will be fine with protein level. However, if a child has very little protein in the diet, you may want to get an assessment of the diet to ensure they have adequate amounts. Signs of protein deficiency include stunted growth, lack of appetite, edema, suppressed immune system, muscle wasting, anxiety, sparse hair, and dry skin.

Grass-fed/Pastured Animal Foods

For protein (like everything else) it's all about quality! Get meat from grass-fed (or pastured) sources. Grass-fed animals have higher levels of anti-inflammatory fats, less inflammatory fats, more vitamin A and D, and more tryptophan (for serotonin and melatonin, both highly implicated in mood and sleep!). (Rule, 2002) (Ponnampalam, 2006). Just as the general public has been misinformed that cholesterol and saturated fats (and even fats in general) are evil, you will find that many nutrition sources propagate the myth that meat is bad. Firstly, I don't think it is, but more importantly all studies done on animal fat and protein are done on conventional cows—not grass-fed, organic, or anything healthy cows. I would agree that commercially raised meat (especially now that cloning and irradiation are allowed) is very bad for you. So it's not that meat is bad but the unhealthy ways the animals are raised. Like us, if animals eat unhealthy food, live in unhealthy conditions, and are injected with unhealthy drugs, they will be unhealthy. We do not want to eat that kind of food.

Organic does not mean the animals eat grass. Organic animals are most often fed organic *grain,* which is inflammatory and not healthy for animals even if it is organic. Therefore, try to buy grass-fed or pastured meat. Try to eat eggs from pastured hens, although these are not easy to find. "Cage-free" is not pastured. Chickens need to be outside getting sunlight and eating bugs in order for their eggs and meat to be optimally healthy. There are also vegetarian sources of protein including nuts, beans, even grains and vegetables have some protein. Consume these plant proteins from organic sources whenever possible.

Vegetarians and soy

Soy is not a good protein source (or substitute for dairy). Soy is very difficult to digest. It irritates the gastrointestinal tract and blocks absorption of vital nutrients such as calcium, magnesium, iron, copper and especially zinc due to phytic acid and oxalates. Soy inhibits thyroid function and cause endocrine disruption in the reproductive hormones of both males and females due to phytoestrogens.

Vegetarian diets often rely upon grains, nuts, beans, and other starches, which can be very inflammatory to the gut. Vegetarian diets often emphasize soy and dairy (two options not tolerated by many with ASD). It can be difficult to be vegetarian when the diet is additionally restricted by food sensitivities. In this case, it can be difficult to get enough protein. I am very respectful of someone's ethical or religious reasons; however, I sometimes ask if parents will reconsider their vegetarian position when eggs, soy, dairy, nuts, and/or beans are excluded. If a child is very low in protein, consider a supplemental protein powder such as rice protein, pea protein, or whey protein. Make sure that the protein powder is a non-hydrolyzed protein so there is no MSG (the only non-hydrolyzed ones I've found are whey-based—not helpful to those on a GFCF diet—Designs for Health sells one). If protein powder will not work, free form amino acids may be necessary or helpful. Five grams of free-form amino acids equals the equivalent of 30 grams of dietary protein. However, be aware the glutamic acid and aspartic acid may be a problem for some with susceptibility to neuroexcitotoxicity (if you're glutamate sensitive).

Carbohydrates

Focus on complex carbohydrates (assuming you are not on the Specific Carbohydrate Diet), such as whole grains (not flour products), vegetables, fruit, and starchy vegetables. These are higher in nutrients and fiber.

Reduce consumption of refined carbohydrates including flour products such as breads, crackers, chips, cookies, and pasta. Refined carbohydrates turn to sugar and feed yeast.

Sugar

Everyone should limit sugar. Those with yeast overgrowth should avoid sugar. Refined sugar, honey, and juices all feed yeast. The exception is on SCD. Because SCD does not allow complex starches in the diet, moderate consumption of fruit and honey appear not to feed yeast. -While you can do some of these allowable sugars on SCD, I would limit them.

For all diets, limit sugar to four to five grams per serving (four grams equals one teaspoon "sugars"). Examples of this amount include two ounces of fruit juice, two teaspoons of dried fruit, 1/3-1/2 apple or peach, a cup of raspberries, ¼ cup of grapes, or one tablespoon of ketchup. Notice, how sweet fruits (grapes) have a much smaller portion size than sour fruits (raspberries). Keep sugar to four of these small servings per day.

While almost all yeast diets agree on avoiding fruit, there are clients who say that fruit does not seem to feed yeast for their child. If a child can only follow a yeast diet by allowing some fruit (not juice except small quantities for supplements), give it a try.

Yeast overgrowth, stress/anxiety (sensory sensitivity), and blood sugar imbalances can cause carbohydrate and sugar cravings. Therefore, if a child has cravings, reduce sugar levels while working on yeast, stress, and balancing blood sugar.

#5 Choosing a Foundational ASD Diet

This section is about removing any offending foods and choosing an "ASD Diet" to begin. Often this involves determining a diet based on what foods your child needs to *avoid*. Most of the ASD diets involve some level of dietary restriction, that is, removing offending foods, whether they are gluten, casein, sugars, grains, or others. The following are foundational diets because they have the largest number of people applying them, with the highest rates of effectiveness. However, any diet can be used as a foundational diet.

- GFCF
- SCD
- BED
- WAP

Each diet is usually applied strictly and independently so as not to introduce principles that could render the diet ineffective. At a point in the future, we may change or combine principles from other diets. In fact, I find that most children do best on and end up with a diet that is a combination of principles from various dietary approaches. However, for this first phase, we want to be able to see results from the diet without interference. This way we can rule out dietary infractions as the cause of the problem, and look for the real cause.

Some parents may already know they need to restrict a diet further to account for allergies or food sensitivities, for example not allow dairy on SCD, or keep corn out of GFCF. If you know you need to do so, you can remove further foods but do not add anything that is not allowed.

Beginning an ASD diet often starts with going GFCF. While many parents start with GFCF, not all do, and not all children benefit from it. Some parents start straight away with SCD, especially when chronic diarrhea is present. BED is another common choice, especially for those with candida as it is one of the more comprehensive and beneficial yeast diets. Nourishing Traditions/Weston A. Price diet (as the name implies) is very nourishing and good for digestion—and doesn't remove any food groups; instead attempts to make commonly problematic foods more digestible.

An important note: anything that creates endorphins, opiates, or drug-like effects on the brain (gluten, casein, phenols, MSG, etc) becomes very addicting. Some children are literally addicted to these foods as though they were drugs. This is why (contrary to what seems to make sense); they often crave the foods that are worst for them. If you cannot remove a food without a complete meltdown, this is a very strong indicator that this is a problem food. This also explains why I'm often met (completely understandably) with fear or disbelief that a parent can remove these foods from the diet because it is the *ONLY* thing the child will eat. I have been told time and time again by parents that they could not believe their child would ever eat vegetables or anything outside of wheat, dairy, and bananas—until they eliminated the food addictions. Only then, little by little, were food choices expanded (sometimes dramatically). So if you are one of those parents who can't believe it is possible to eliminate these foods, you are not alone, you are not the first to feel this way, and you can be successful.

Gluten-free and Casein-Free

> *Does your child crave milk?*
> *Does your child only eat wheat and dairy foods?*
> *Does your child have constipation?*
> *Does your child seem spacey after consuming gluten or casein, and agitated before?*
> *Are you just beginning to look at diet for the first time?*
> *Is your child a very picky eater?*

According to parents (Autism Research Institute survey), a gluten- and casein-free diet is helpful for 65% of children with ASD even though a food sensitivity panel may or may not have shown a reaction to these foods. Therefore, I typically recommend a gluten- and casein-free trial period—often starting the diet by removing first one, then the other. The questions above are a few I consider when deciding whether to try GFCF.

Many practitioners are so strict about the need to implement GFCF, that they often ignore the feedback from parents. Many times, I have had clients tell me that the diet made no difference or their child can do either wheat or dairy just fine. After speaking with them I realized that the problem is not with the parent, it is the diet. The diet has received great promotion, as it deserves and which we need as it is helpful for a great number of children. However, the diet does not work for all. There also appears to be some percentage of children, who do well initially on GFCF, and then regress after a period of time—even when they have followed it strictly and not added other possible offending foods. We don't know why this happens. My advice: give the diet a good, wholehearted implementation and trial. Seek help from an experienced parent or professional if problems arise, progress is not seen, or regression happens. If the diet is truly not working, try something else.

can be very effective if it is followed with awareness. For more on when to use this diet see *ASD Diet Options*. See Appendix V for a more thorough list of foods that contain gluten and casein and substitutes that are gluten- and casein-free, and a list of hidden sources of gluten.

Specific Carbohydrate Diet:

> *Does your child have chronic diarrhea?*
> *Does your child have an inflamed gut, maybe even been on steroids?*
> *Have you tried GFCF to no avail?*
> *Does your child have trouble digesting grains?*
> *Does your child eat meat?*
> *Does your child have a nut allergy or attend a school with a no nut policy? (If so this diet may not be for you)*
> *Does your child have a problem with ammonia? (If so, this diet is high in protein and may not be right)*

SCD is the second most common foundational diet with 66% of parents saying it was beneficial for their child (ARI ratings). It is very helpful for those who have inflammatory bowel conditions and chronic diarrhea, although it can help constipation too. If you do not have the ability to use nuts in the diet, either because the child is allergic, or because the school has a no nut policy, this diet can be very difficult. It is very helpful for dysbiosis that creates inflammation in the gut.

For more on when to use this diet and for resources to implement the diet see *ASD Diet Options*. For SCD compliant foods see Appendix VII. For more on the details of implementing SCD see *Breaking the Vicious Cycle* by Elaine Gottschall and www.breakingtheviciouscycle.info. See Resources for more on SCD.

Body Ecology Diet

> *Does you child have persistent candida?*
> *Does your child have harmful bacteria in the gut?*
> *Does your child have bad smelling stool or gas?*
> *Does your child sometimes act drunk, spacey or have maniacal laughter?*
> *Does your child seem itchy or yeasty in any "moist" areas of the body like elbows, knees, or crotch?*
> *Does your child eat vegetables?*

If you child has candida this diet is one of the best. However, it requires that the child eats vegetables as the food combining aspect allows meat with vegetables and starches with vegetables but not meat and starch together. Vegetables and alkalizing foods are emphasized, as are fermented foods. If a child is picky and does not have a varied diet, this diet will be difficult.

For more on when to use this diet and for resources to implement the diet see *ASD Diet Options*.

Nourishing Traditions/Weston A. Price

> *Are you uncomfortable or uninterested in restricting any foods to start?*
> *Do you want to start with increasing levels of nourishment?*
> *Does your child digest fat well?*
> *Does your child eat animal food?*
> *Does your child seem to have a certain tolerance for milk and/or wheat (seems to be able to consume certain forms without a problem)?*
> *Do you have access to foods such as pastured meat and raw milk?*
> *Would you like a diet that can be implemented for the whole family?*

This is a great diet for anyone looking for a good, nourishing diet. It is helpful for digestion as the preparation techniques make the food much more digestible. The fermented foods are wonderful for yeast and the gut. This diet incorporates many solid principles of nutrition. Foods may need to be removed later but it will get the family started on a healthy diet with a lot of nutrients that has the most flavor and variety of the bunch.

For more on when to use this diet and for resources to implement the diet see *ASD Diet Options*.

Tips for the First Step of ASD Diet Implementation

Consider implementing as many dietary changes for the whole family as possible. This would be a worthwhile step if all family members (who general share genetic backgrounds) seem to suffer from problems I listed in Part I of the book. Furthermore, we never want a child with an ASD to feel punished by these dietary changes, and including the rest of the family as much as possible reduces the possibility of these feelings arising.

My clients' strategies vary by family:

- Some do not allow any of the restricted foods in the house because the child can climb on the counter and get into them.
- Others keep them in the house but have a lock (literally) on the refrigerator or cupboards.
- Some have a well hidden stash for certain family members.
- Others only enjoy non-permissible foods when they are out of the house and/or the child that is sensitive is not present.

Start any diet by adding new foods before you remove old foods. This will provide more food options and familiarity with these new foods for a smooth transition. Often people implement the diets gradually; although some find it easier to do it all at one. Ultimately, there is not correct way. However, slowly is a little easier on the body, but sometimes a little more difficult on the psyche. When there is gray area it can be confusing for the child, or he might decide to just move from one food addiction to another if you don't remove them all together.

Make a plan. Put together a list of acceptable and not acceptable foods for the particular diet. Find some recipes that you think your child might like—maybe something similar to what he already likes. Come up with some meal options. Create a meal plan, daily, or weekly menu with shopping items. Search out a good source for quality food and specialty items such as a co-op, local market or natural food store. Try cooking or baking a few foods and see how things come out.

It often takes some time to get used to the nuances of a new diet. But trust me, you will get into the swing of things and it will be much faster and easier.

While typically people follow this foundational diet for six months, you can move to the next step before that. Generally, I recommend that both you and your child have settled into an ASD diet. That is, the parents know what foods to give, the child will eat the foods and has enough quantity and variety, and there are no noticeable negative food reactions. Once these criteria are met to your comfort, you can move on to the next step. If the diet does not seem to be helping very much, consider adding *Step #6* and remove food intolerances. If you believe you've addressed all food intolerances and are seeing a big regression, you'll want to seek assistance on implementation of diet or switch to another foundational diet.

#6 Addressing Food Intolerances: Food Sensitivities and Phenols

Food intolerances are any foods someone cannot tolerate. Intolerances may include food sensitivities, phenols, amines, lectins and more. First let us address food sensitivities and phenols. We will talk about amines and lectins in the next two sections.

Food Sensitivities/Allergies

There are two main types of allergenic reactions: IgE (food allergies) and IgG (food sensitivities). Both of these kinds of allergens are important to eliminate from the diet. An IgE reaction is acute and much more obvious than an IgG reaction. A food allergy reaction might include hives, sneezing/running nose, or anaphylactic shock (as when the throat swells closed from eating a peanut). As these reactions are more immediate and obvious, they are typically easier to recognize.

The IgG antibody reaction is what we have been talking about when we say food sensitivity. It is a slower response that could take hours or days to appear, making it difficult to detect. The most common food sensitivities (in order of highest first) are: gluten, casein, soy, corn, eggs, peanuts, citrus, chocolate, and cane sugar. The second tier of food sensitivities include: tree nuts, seeds, beef, yeast, and tomatoes. However, you can have a food sensitivity to anything. IgG reactions can cause gut inflammation and cause further sensitivities to develop. In addition to diarrhea, constipation, aggression, lethargy, and the myriad of symptoms we see with food sensitivities, also look for extreme cravings or self-limiting to only certain foods. I have had clients who were so addicted to the opiates and endorphins that they could not get back to sleep in the middle of the night until having some milk or toast. I have also had clients (adults and kids) raid the refrigerator in the middle of the night and eat an entire block of cheese or box of ice cream bars. This is not common with all food sensitivities, but it is a "classic sign" if you have this behavior happening. This is why the following two tests are very helpful in uncovering these sensitivities.

Assessing food sensitivities

The two most common ways to determine food sensitivities are the antibody blood test (see assessments in the Impact of Nutrients section) and an elimination diet. The elimination diet, while more cost effective than the laboratory testing, is much more tedious. If you can notice reactions in your child, the elimination is the ultimate detection method and "gold standard," as the child's reaction through diet is the best indicator of what is actually happening to the child, and the blood test can give false positive and negative results.

If your child has received an allergy test from the doctor that was a skin scratch test, this will only test for IgE allergies. Parents OFTEN tell me that there doctor said their child does not have an "allergy" to wheat based on this test. While what they said is technically correct, we are looking for a food sensitivity, not allergy, and sensitivities cannot be tested with a scratch test.

Two blood tests used to determine IgG antibody reactions to food sensitivities are the ELISA and RAST. While both are similar, ELISA appears to be more sensitive and is used more commonly by doctors. I know some doctors that prefer to run both tests to compare results. Another test to consider if the IgG does not yield helpful results is the LEAP test at nowleap.com. It tests for cell mediated response and tests food additives/chemicals as well as foods. Neither test is perfect. If you haven't eaten a food in a long time, a reaction will not typically show in the result (and you will get a false negative). While I find the LEAP test intriguing, I have not seen enough results to recommend it instead of the IgG, which is used by most physicians and has a lot more clinical data. However, if you suspect food chemicals or amines may be a problem, LEAP is a good test to try as it is the only one I know of that can address these.

As it can be common for children with ASD to have a dozen or more food sensitivities, some of them unexpected foods such as rice, these lab tests can provide a good place to start. One word of caution though, 10-15% of the time these tests produce false positives or negatives, so the ultimate authority is dietary testing (food elimination/provocation)—testing the food to determine any reaction from the child. Additionally, don't rely completely on the number scale. If the test shows a small reaction to a food (VL or 1+) this could be just as significant reaction as a 4+. The tests just give good guidelines and places to start the experimentation process. Additionally, if a food does not show up at all but you experience symptoms upon consumption and relief upon removal, then go with the experience and not the test result. If dozens of foods show up as positive on the test the approach is trickier, as it often not possible to eliminate every food completely. I typically approach this latter situation with a combination of food eliminations, rotation diet, and enzymes.

If reactions are difficult to spot, another way is to follow the above instructions for the diet and use pulse (heart rate) as a measure of intolerance. If the pulse is elevated 10-15 beats/minute immediately after a food is consumed (or sometimes even held in hand), this is an indication of intolerance. This leads us to the idea of muscle testing. This is where someone puts their arm out to the side and another person pushes it down—the weakness or strength of the arm indicates the person's tolerance or benefit from the food or substance. For a child, you can be a "surrogate" and do the muscle testing for them. Some have great success with muscle testing and become believers in energy work. People even use various forms of energy work to not only assess but *clear* food sensitivities: Bioset, NAET, and a form of energy work I do called Bioenergy Balancing are a few I have heard good things about (See Resources).

Food sensitivities and infants

Please note that food sensitivities can be created in utero when a mother with food intolerances eats those foods during pregnancy (or possibly when a mother eats foods that baby is sensitive to because of sensitivities the father has passed on). Additionally, IgG antibodies can pass into the breast milk. This is strongly believed to be one major reason for colic. Think back into your history and whether your child had a lot of digestive problems when nursing: colic, thrush, eczema, or digestive/elimination problems. It's possible you and/or your child have had these food sensitivities for a while.

Here are a few things to think of if you are planning more children in the future. For mothers and/or their babies who have food sensitivities, a breastfeeding mother will want to avoid all food sensitivities in her diet. For mothers who cannot breast feed, formula becomes an agonizing decision as these mothers understand the benefits of breastfeeding and that the alternatives typically involve introducing cow's milk or soymilk—two non-ideal solutions as they are the most common sensitivities and soy has a separate list of negative reasons not to use it. I never recommend soy formula. Sally Fallon has some "lifesavers" for formulas in her book *Nourishing Traditions*. I love these recipes because they cover the full range of needs from a fortifying standard formula, to making your own formula from whatever milk you are the most comfortable with (organic, raw, goat's, etc.), and a non-dairy based formula (using liver and broth) for those who are highly casein sensitive.

Salicylates/Phenols

If the parent still suspects further problem foods and is confident they do not arise from one of the food sensitivities above, test results have revealed poor detoxification and sulfation, or the child has a reaction to the substances listed below, I would consider phenols as the culprit. In this situation, I would try the Feingold Diet.

The Feingold diet involves eliminating food additive phenols, such as artificial colors (such as "FD&C Red #2," "Yellow #5," "U.S. Certified Color," "Color Added," etc.), artificial flavors (including "vanillin," "artificial flavoring," "flavoring,") and preservatives (such as BHA, BHT, and TBHQ). Hopefully you have already eliminated these in step #1. If step #1 hasn't been taken at this point, that would become your first priority. Then you can try eliminating the most reactive foods containing salicylates—those eliminated on the Feingold Diet. A full list of phenols and salicylates eliminated in stage 1 of the Feingold Diet can be found in Appendix XII; some of them include apples, grapes, cucumbers, oranges, bananas, aspirin, benzoates (sodium benzoate, benzoic acid), and sulfating agents (including sulfur dioxide, sodium sulfite, sodium bisulfate, etc.). After eliminating these foods and additives for four weeks, you may re-introduce the salicylate foods back, one at a time. Observe the response for five days and record the results. If you feel they are non-offending items, you can add them back permanently and you can go on to the next food for testing (Hersey, 2002). If you have already determined foods that the child is sensitive to, do not add these foods back even if they are "allowed" in the Feingold Diet. Again, never add back artificial ingredients and food additives—they are terrible for everyone.

I use a combination of physical, biochemical, behavioral, and cognitive sign/symptoms to get a sense as to whether reducing phenols and addressing sulfation may be helpful. Reactions to foods and substances are the first things I look for—any obvious reaction to artificial ingredients and other strong chemical phenols like Tylenol. Next, I look for unusual or extreme cravings for natural salicylates like apples and grapes. A few examples that I have heard in my practice from parents should help illustrate this: inconsolable tantrum after consumption of colored sprinkles on birthday cake, extreme aggression from consumption of candy sweetened with grape juice, and consumption of only apple juice as a beverage.

Feingold is a good place to start, but only eliminates certain salicylates. If you need further refinement, Failsafe is a further restriction of phenols and phenol-like substances. See Appendix VII for further details to help determine sensitivity and how to address phenols. If you suspect faulty sulfation and phenol intolerance, go to the section discussing phenol protocol, I have created a three pronged approach: (1) Reduce phenolic foods and chemicals, (2) help break down the phenols better, and (3) improve processing of phenols by supplementing the building blocks of sulfation/methylation. In this step, start with removing phenols. The third piece, which supplements may or may not be helpful, depends on individual chemistry and is tackled in steps #3 and #10.

#7 Evolving the Diet: Nutrition Boosters

Anywhere along the process you can begin to increase nutrient density and digestibility of foods in the diet. I've added it at this point (later in the holistic approach) because often "ideal nutrition" is not our initial goal. Most parents get the toxic foods out first: food additives, food allergies and sensitivities, and phenols. Once they feel they can begin to incorporate these new changes, they start this step. Other parents, especially the ones who start with the Nourishing Traditions/Weston A. Price diet, start with this step from the beginning. There is no specific rationale or need to wait until this step in the process.

You can get good nutrients in the diet through several means:
- Increasing the quality of the foods your child already eats.
- Sneaking nutrients in the diet, even with picky eaters.
- Making foods more digestible for better nutrient absorption by using traditional cooking methods such as soaking and fermenting. (Grandma did know best!)

Increasing the Quality of the Foods Your Child Already Eats

One of the simplest things to do, especially for picky eaters, is to start with foods they already enjoy such as eggs, oatmeal, fruit or vegetables, and beef or chicken. Most of the time a child will not notice the switch to a higher quality, while you get the added nutrients into him or her. Moreover, these foods have so much more flavor. These principles of quality include:

- Grass-fed
- Organic
- Vine ripened
- Fresh from farmer

As we previously discussed (in Step #4, *Diet Basics*), grass-fed animal proteins and fats are far superior in good/essential fats and fat-soluble vitamins. Additionally, grass-fed animals are not fed inflammatory grain—one of the reasons I strongly believe people develop a food sensitivity to animal products. Commercial meat can be inflammatory. For this reason, switching to grass-fed beef and lamb, pastured chickens and eggs, and pastured dairy products (if not casein-free) are simple changes any family can make. The chicken, eggs, and dairy are far more delicious, without being "strange." Grass-fed beef on the other hand, may take some time getting used to as the fatty acids make it stronger in flavor.

Organic and vine ripened are also important. Organic is important because of the increase in nutrients and decrease in pesticides. I know it is not always possible or economically feasible to buy organic for everything. The following is a chart from the Environmental Working Group on the 12 dirtiest and cleanest produce to give you an idea of what to make sure you find organic and what is okay to buy conventional when you have to. The Environmental Working Group is an incredible resource for making healthy decisions for your family. Their website is www.ewg.org/

Highest pesticides - Buy these organic	**Lowest in pesticides**
Peaches	Onions
Apples	Avocado
Sweet bell peppers	Sweet Corn (Frozen)
Celery	Pineapples
Nectarines	Mango
Strawberries	Sweet Peas (Frozen)
Cherries	Asparagus
Lettuce	Kiwi
Grapes (Imported)	Bananas
Pears	Cabbage
Spinach	Broccoli
Potatoes	Eggplant

Vine ripened produce has more nutrients, more essential sugars (these are good, similar to glyconutrient supplements), and less phenols. Conventional farms pick fruits and vegetables green for less spoilage and ripened on the truck or by gassing the produce (an unhealthy process) to ripen. In the last several days of ripening on the vine or tree, a number of nutrients are transferred from the plant to the fruit. It is very important to get vine ripened whenever possible.

142

Go to the farmer's market or get to know a farmer. Often small farms do not use pesticides but have not paid the fees to be "certified organic." By going to the farmer (at the farm, farmers' market, or through community supported agriculture—CSA), you can fairly easily meet the criteria above. This is a great way to support the farmer and get high quality food at prices you can afford. Straight from the farmer ensures the food is fresher, has more energy and nutrients intact, and in most cases, is vine ripened. CSA's are typically a box delivery service where you receive a weekly or bimonthly box of food that is locally grown and in season—there are those straight from the farmer that I recommend, or those that have a middleman organizing it.

Grass-fed meat is available at some grocery stores, but pastured eggs typically are not. Also, you can often get better prices and quality if you go to through a farmer or buy in with a co-op. The Weston A. Price Foundation is a great resource to find good sources of meat and produce. There are chapters worldwide and members have wonderful information on food sources.

By increasing the quality of the foods your child already enjoys, you will boost nutrition without him or her even noticing.

Sneaking Nutrients in the Diet, even with Picky Eaters.

There are many ways to get more nutrients in the diet. For some children these foods discussed below are already in their diet and will be simple to implement. In other cases, we will want to start slow and find ways to sneak them in.

Nutrient-Dense Foods

Nutrient-dense foods are foods rich in vitamins and minerals—they are packed with nutrients, maximizing nutrients in each calorie. Here is a great list of foods to add to the diet and what nutrients they are high in:

- **Sweet potatoes**: fiber, beta carotene, B6, pantothenic acid (B5), potassium
- **Eggs, meat, and animal fat from pastured hens/animals**: B12, vitamin A, B vitamins, vitamin D, vitamin E, selenium, calcium, iodine, zinc, iron, EPA, DHA, CLA (Conjugated linoleic acid)
- **Bone broth/stock**: calcium, magnesium, phosphorus, silicon, sulfur, chondroitin and glucosamine sulfates, trace minerals, gelatin
- **Beans and legumes**: folic acid, B6, potassium, magnesium, zinc, iron
- **Whole grains**: selenium, vitamin E, magnesium, B6
- **Leafy greens**: calcium, vitamin C, folic acid, beta carotene, vitamin A, magnesium, iron
- **Nettles** (can make a tea): calcium, magnesium, potassium
- **Blackstrap molasses**: iron, magnesium, selenium, potassium, calcium
- **Nuts and seeds**: calcium, magnesium, iron, zinc, B6, vitamin E, folic acid
- **Hemp seeds**: GLA, omega-3, vitamin E, methionine, cysteine, L-arginine. Arginine is important for childhood growth and reduces high ammonia levels; however, not good for active herpes infection. Hemp contains all essential amino acids to form a complete protein like meat.
- **Kombu and seaweed**: calcium, magnesium, iron
- **Organic liver**: iron, vitamin C, B12, folic acid, beta carotene, vitamin A

The following is the list of foods above with some ideas on how to incorporate these foods in the diet, in addition to eating them whole.

Food	Getting it into the diet
Sweet potatoes	Make fries. Cook, puree and add to smoothies, meatballs, or tomato sauce.
Eggs	Scrambled and eaten or added to homemade fried rice. Soaked into bread for french toast.
Meat	Meatballs, meat patties, in spaghetti sauce
Bone broth	Used to make soup. Cook rice or other grain in broth. Add a splash to tomato sauce. Even cook pasta in to absorb a few nutrients.
Beans and legumes	Cook, puree and add to soup or sauce to thicken. Added whole to soups.
Whole grains	Make baked goods with whole grains. Cook whole grains similar to rice and eat as side dish. Add to soup.
Leafy greens	Cook, puree, and add to meatballs or tomato sauce. Add to vegetable juices. Simmer in bone or mineral broth, and then remove.
Nettles	Simmer in bone or mineral broth, and then remove. Use dried as a tea.
Nuts and seeds	Nut milks, nut butter, nut flours.
Hemp seeds	Sprinkle on toast with nut butter. Add to finished quinoa (grain) dish.
Blackstrap molasses	Add to muffins. Use as sweetener in oatmeal. Only need a little. Hot water with one tablespoon molasses with a squeeze of honey, great for iron absorption.
Kombu and seaweed	Simmer in bone or mineral broth. Add to cooking soup, grain, or bean.
Organic liver	Blend in food processor and add small amount to meatballs or patties. Make chopped liver or pate if child likes spreads.

Mineral-rich Broths and Stocks

Broths and stocks are great ways to increase consumption of highly absorbable nutrients. Broths and stocks (I think of stocks as bone-based) can be made vegetarian or with animal meat and bones.

For a great mineral broth, you can use potatoes, carrots, celery, parsley, seaweed, and or any vegetable, green, or herb. This very nutrient-dense vegetable broth can be used in several ways. You can use the broth as a base in a prepare soup. You can cook grains or beans in a broth to absorb the nutrients. You can even drink as a tea. I often take *Nourishing Traditions'* Potassium Broth recipe and add seaweed, nettles and other vegetables.

Meat stocks (bone broths) are traditionally used by most native cultures as a way to nourish the sick, elderly, and mothers after childbirth. Grandma's old remedy of chicken soup when you're sick was based on a great deal of truth. The bones (of chicken, beef, lamb or whatever you like) add calcium, magnesium and potassium into the broth. The addition of vegetables to these stocks adds electrolytes. *Nourishing Traditions* by Sally Fallon and the Weston A. Price Foundation website (WestonAPrice.org) have recipes for making a traditional broth.

The natural gelatin in bone broths is wonderfully rejuvenative for digestion. The gelatin contains high levels of glycine and proline, which help heal the gut. Glycine also helps with sleep, detoxification of environmental toxins, and the formation of glutathione. Proline aids the formation of connective tissue in skin, the gut, and ligaments. Bone broths (like raw foods described earlier) are hydrophilic colloidals, drawing water to enhance digestion.

Gelatin is broken down by DPP-IV, an enzyme discussed previously for its important role in the digestion of peptides. It is important to have enough of this enzyme and I often recommend that my clients take an enzyme with DPP-IV in it, such as Houston Enzymes, Kirkman, or Klaire Labs.

Be aware, gelatin contains free glutamate, which is potentially problematic for glutamate sensitive people. However, this natural gelatin seems to not be as problematic as the free glutamate that is in commercial gelatin. Russell Blaylock, M.D., author of *Excitotoxins: The Taste That Kills*, in an email exchange with my research assistant mentioned he believes natural gelatin functions differently and is most likely not problematic for most. This may be because the extraction process of commercial gelatin is much different than that of making stocks. Most people are fine with this natural gelatin and find it healing. However, if you are really glutamate sensitive you'll want to pay special attention to whether you have a reaction to the gelatin in stocks.

One more comment on the amino acids in stocks. According to Sally Fallon, arginine and glycine can spare protein, allowing the body to utilize more fully the complete proteins that are found in other sources (Fallon, 2001). This can be advantageous for those children who do not eat much protein.

Minerals are absorbed in ionic form. If they are not in ionic form when consumed, they are ionized in the gut as salts dissolving into their two components (or chelates) releasing their key elements. Mineral-rich bone broths have all of the macrominerals—sodium, chloride, calcium, magnesium, phosphorus, potassium and sulfur available in ready-to-use ionized form as a true electrolyte solution. Vegetable broths are also ionic. Additionally, unrefined sea salt and crystal salt (such as a Himalayan crystal salt) can supply these minerals in ionic form and are therefore excellent to add to the broth. See "Salt" in the "Impact of Nutrients" section for further information on this.

Juicing

Juicing vegetables is a way to get great concentrations of nutrients without all of the bulk of the fiber. Chlorophyll and phytonutrients are plentiful in vegetable juices.

Juicing works well for children who like liquids, juices, and smoothies. You want to drink freshly made juice immediately, within minutes if possible. Whatever is not consumed immediately should be placed in a glass container (to the top to minimize exposure to oxygen) and then stored with an airtight lid in the refrigerator.

Juicing the anti-inflammatory vegetables, root vegetables, and fruits from *Step #11 Immune Support* is a great way to go. Avoid too many sweet vegetables (like carrots) and fruits. Using celery, cucumber, fennel, ginger, and green apple is a good place to start.

When buying a juicer there are several types. Masticating juicers operates at a slower speed and chews the fibers and breaks up the cells of vegetables and fruits. This gives you more fiber, enzymes, vitamins and trace minerals; however, it also heats up the juice and can destroy some of the enzymes and nutrients. These types of juicers can also blend up frozen bananas into a natural banana-only "ice cream" and make nut butters. Centrifugal juicers first grind the fruit and vegetables then push them through the strainer by spinning at a very high rpm. These yield more juice and don't heat the juice. Triturating juicers (twin gear) are less common and twice the price of other juicers. The two step process, first crushing the fruits and vegetables, then pressing the juice allows for more fiber, enzymes, vitamins and trace minerals and can juice wheatgrass—something the other juicers cannot do. There is no one juicer that's best—much of it depends on your needs and budget. I have a centrifugal because it meets my basic needs and doesn't heat the juice. However, many love the Champion juicer (masticating), and the banana "ice cream" is delicious and a great treat on SCD. Online is often the best place to buy one.

Sneaking in Nutrients

As you can, start adding and even sneaking nutrients into the food. To summarize some of the ways to best get more nutrients in the diet:

- Cook and puree vegetables. Freeze in ice cube trays and add to smoothies.
- Cook and puree any vegetables and add to meatballs, meat patties, meatloaf, or pasta sauce.
- Cook grains or even pasta in homemade broth.
- Nettles can be consumed as a tea, or added to a homemade broth
- Add kombu or other sea vegetable to cooking grains, soups, tomato sauce, even boiling pasta.
- Add a little blackstrap molasses as a sweetener.

Soaking and Fermenting

Soaking and fermenting "seeds"

By "seeds" I mean grains, beans, nuts and seeds—anything that is the seed of a plant—not just seeds such as sunflower seeds. Traditional cultures prepared their grains (seeds) much differently than we do. The Weston A. Price foundation's website (westonaprice.org) references Keith Steinkraus' book, *Handbook of Indigenous Fermented Foods*, where he states that in Sub-Saharan Africa (similar to most traditional cultures), "Preparation 'at the homestead' begins with washing the grains, then steeping them in water for 24 to 72 hours. The grain is drained and the water discarded. The smooth paste... undergo[es] further fermentation." Native cultures knew that soaking and fermenting grains kept people healthy. Soaking seeds in a moist, slightly acidic and warm environment mimics the seeds' natural germination process in the soil. Only when the phytates are broken down can the seed release its enzymes and nutrients for growth.

These preparations make the foods much more nutritious than modern grain preparations. Soaking, and particularly fermenting, grains, beans and other "seeds" (grains, beans, nuts and seeds) increases mineral availability, increases vitamin content, predigests starches, and neutralizes enzyme inhibitors, phytic acid, oxalates, and lectins. Interestingly, soy is very high in phytates and lectins making it very difficult to digest. This is why in Asia they traditionally soaked and fermented soy for weeks if not months—a practice not used in soy products sold in North America.

Enzyme inhibitors inhibit a variety of natural digestive enzymes—pancreatic inhibitors, protease inhibitors, and trypsin inhibitors—and are very problematic for children on the autistic spectrum. These enzyme inhibitors put a strain on digestion, but fortunately, they can be inactivated with soaking and fermentation. Because of the effects on the pancreatic enzymes, it is especially helpful and important for individuals with blood sugar regulation problems such as hypoglycemia and diabetes, to soak any grains they consume.

Oxalates, phytates, and lectins are particularly problematic, evidenced by the fact that there are numerous diets out there to address them. We know from parental experience that many children on the spectrum have trouble with oxalates, and parents are using the low oxalate diet as a way of addressing them (with another group trying to address the issue through supplementation). No grain diets—SCD, Paleo, GAPS—address oxalates, phytates and lectins to some extent by removing the source (grain) high in these substances. There is a newer group of parents looking at addressing lectins by inactivating them through soaking and fermenting, and also using supplements to render them harmless to the body. http://health.groups.yahoo.com/group/lectins_in_autism/ is the yahoo group looking specifically at this.

Phytates (or phytic acid) are present on the surface of all seeds. Phytates block mineral absorption in the gut—particularly zinc, calcium, magnesium, and iron—four minerals often in short supply in those with ASD. Phytates are inflammatory to the gut. Additionally, phytates can adversely impact brain function by binding to zinc and calcium—important nutrients for the brain. Digestive enzymes containing phytase, an enzyme that breaks down phytates, are frequently used with ASD, as many in the field are aware of the challenge with digestion and mineral absorption. While this can help, soaking and fermenting are a simple and more effective way to address phytates. Soaking and fermenting can address things that enzymes can't.

Oxalates, which are not broken down by enzymes, can be removed and neutralized by soaking. Oxalates, like phytates, block absorption of zinc, calcium, magnesium, and iron and are very inflammatory to the gut. Additionally, they can create pain throughout the body.

Lectins also cause inflammation in the gut. They too are resistant to digestive enzymes, but can be broken down through soaking and/or fermentation. Lectins damage the gut by binding to the intestinal wall, at times creating leaky gut that allows lectins and bacteria into the blood stream and the body. Once in the body, lectins can bind to cells on any organ and create inflammation and damage by causing an autoimmune reaction. In a study on gut integrity (and vitamin A), the author makes a reference to lectins, "Food antigens, possibly dietary lectins, can have potent antinutritional properties, influencing the structure and function of both enterocytes and lymphocytes. Lectins are glycoproteins that occur in common dietary staples such as cereal grains and legumes. Lectins in general can bind to the surface glycans on gut brush border epithelial cells, causing damage to the base of the villi, disarrangement of the cyto- skeleton, increasing endocytosis, and shortening of microvilli. The structural changes induced by lectins upon epithelial cells elicit functional changes, including increased permeability, which may then facilitate the passage of undergraded antigens and pathogenic bacteria into the system circulation" (Thurnham, 2000)

Fermentation has been show to be very effective in breaking down the lectins. In fact, in a study done in Italy, celiac patients were able to consume sourdough bread made with a mixture of wheat and other grains that had been fermented by lactobacilli. The fermentation process broke down the inflammatory compounds to such an extent that the celiac patients were able to eat it without responding to the gluten (Di Cagno, 2004).

While I'm not suggesting everyone go out and eat sourdough wheat bread, I believe that using these soaking and fermenting methods with grains that are tolerated is a great way to make them even more digestible and less inflammatory, possibly even allowing some people tolerate otherwise problematic foods. There are supplements that are being used to "soak up" the lectins. One is Lectin Lock, the other is n-acetyl glucosamine. Some parents are having good results; however, these are not widely used yet.

Depending on the seed, there are various ways to do prepare it traditionally. While it does take some forethought, the process is quite simple and the time commitment minimal. While I often use a couple tablespoons of whey in the water covering the grain to create an acidic environment to ferment grains particularly oats and wheat, those with casein sensitivity can use lemon juice to create a similar acidity. Additionally, water alone can be used too. *Nourishing Traditions* does a good job of explaining the process of soaking and fermenting. However, be aware that beans soak better in an alkaline environment—a healthy pinch of baking soda.

Nut milks: One of my favorite uses for soaked nuts is making nut milk. By soaking nuts you dramatically increase digestibility and assimilation of nutrients over commercially bought nut milks. You also have more flexibility to make milks with other nuts/seeds to support rotation diets and for those sensitive to the standard almond milk. There is also more "life force" energy in fresh food than boxed food. For example, making your nut milk as opposed to buying it will really increase the digestibility and therefore the nutrients and energy available in the beverage. Recipes for soaking and making nut milk are available on my website (www.HealthfulLiving.org). Choose what you have the time to make based on the diet and time available. If you have the time, it will be worth your while.

The fact that for the most part we eat unsoaked/unsprouted/unfermented grains, nuts, and soy is why I believe so many people have trouble with these foods—they are indigestible without these important processes, and these processes are missing from modern food processing and home preparation. In the "old days" all cultures had their own soaking and fermenting methods; obviously we've lost, and would do well to regain, that ancient wisdom.

Begin to soak or ferment grains, nuts, and beans. These are immensely beneficial changes to make in the diet. Digestion is enhanced greatly and food reactions often diminish. These methods are worth the extra effort. Start with one the food at a time to try this process on.

Fermented foods

Fermented foods are another enzyme-rich food source. Fermented foods such as yogurt, kefir, raw sauerkraut, and kombucha are very important for good health. The good bacteria (and good yeast in some cases) are beneficial to the digestive tract, crowd out and kill bad yeast and pathogenic bacteria, and increase enzyme and nutrient content in the food. Some fermentations are bacteria-only fermentations such as sauerkraut and yogurt. Others contain a combination of bacteria and yeast (that kills candida) such as kefir and kombucha.

Those that follow traditional diets use fermented foods as an essential part of good nutrition. This is because for many generations, fermenting food was our only way to keep food fresh without refrigeration and eat vegetables during cold winters where vegetables could not be grown. As such, we ate fermented foods daily, which ensured the intestinal tract was populated with good bacteria and we were provided with adequate nutrients. Today most of us eat zero fermented foods. A great book for recipes for making fermented foods is *Wild Fermentation* by Sandor Ellix Katz.

Fermented dairy: Many on the ASD spectrum cannot eat dairy so fermented dairy such as yogurt and kefir may not be a possibility for those people. Some of those on the SCD and those who have cleaned up the gut, often do well with homemade goat's yogurt or homemade raw yogurt. Homemade yogurt is much different—commercial yogurt has milk solids added making it more difficult to digest because of extra lactose. You can make yogurt at home with a yogurt maker, a yogurt starter (make sure it's a non-dairy starter), and a choice of milk (dairy and non-dairy): whole milk, raw milk, goat's milk, and nut milk. Kefir, most commonly made from milk, is made with kefir grains or a powdered kefir starter. The powdered kefir starter such as from BodyEcology.com is easier to experiment with as you have many tries to get it right (although not casein-free). The kefir grains are reusable as they continue to multiple as long as you keep them fermenting, so it's more cost effective in the long run. Most grains were likely grown in dairy initially.

See the section on SCD that follows for more information on raw dairy and its many benefits.

Water kefir: Young green coconut water kefir is a great alternative for those who cannot tolerate dairy, and even for those who can. You get the benefit of the kefir cultures without the casein. Kefir is a culture of beneficial bacteria and yeast. The yeast in kefir kills harmful yeast such as candida albicans and, as such, can be very helpful for many ASD kids.. The taste of young coconut water kefir is pretty good and many kids like it and will drink it. Unfortunately, this drink is not made commercially and has to be made by hand. I have to admit it is a bit time consuming and touchy to make; however, if you can't find the coconuts or do not have the patience, you can buy the coconut water packaged (while maybe not as fresh and pure as straight from coconuts, it's a good option). The other thing to be noted is that some people have sensitivity to coconut. You can find the recipe for coconut kefir in *The Body Ecology Diet* by Donna Gates and on her website www.bodyecologydiet.com. However, be aware—the Body Ecology starter contains casein. You can buy water kefir grains online that are never cultured in dairy and use them instead of the BED culture starter. The "grains" (not really grains) are reusable and more cost effective. The water kefir grains are different than dairy kefir grains.

Fermented vegetables: Raw sauerkraut, cultured vegetables and kim chi are types of fermented vegetables. All cultured foods are sour, a product of the acidic bacteria. You can really experience this sour taste with raw sauerkraut. While it took me a while to fully enjoy it, it grows on you and the sour flavor becomes very enjoyable. Some children love sauerkraut and its sour taste; others (especially those who don't like vegetables) will not touch it. Because of the substantial benefits from cultured vegetables, it really is worth the effort to try them with your child. In some locations, you can by raw cultured vegetables in natural food stores. For other people, where raw cultured vegetables are not available and for a much more cost-effective solution, you can make your own. It's actually quite simple. For some of my favorite recipes see *Wild Fermentation* by Sandor Katz.

Kombucha is a cultured food we don't hear too much about, but it is catching on very quickly. It is my favorite of the cultured foods. It is delicious and kids often love it! Kombucha is often misclassified as "mushroom tea" leading people to believe it is some sort of mushroom boiled and made into a tea. This is not the case. It is a brew of sweetened black or green tea that is fermented with a culture of bacteria and yeast. The bacteria and yeast feed on the sugar and convert it into beneficial components that help with digestion, detoxification, immune function, and cellular metabolism. It almost seems unbelievable when you see all of the problems it can help address, including: constipation, candida, digestive disturbances, immune system problems like AIDS, cancer, headaches, and a variety of heart issues.

The beneficial yeast and bacteria in kombucha compete with and inhibit pathogenic microbes such as strains of candida, staphylococcus, e. coli, salmonella, listeria, and helicobacterpylori, as one study articulates, "Kombucha may be a healthful beverage in view of its anti-microbial activity against a range of pathogenic bacteria. This may promote immunity and general well being. It is recommended that Kombucha be consumed at 33 g/L total acid, 7 g/L acetic acid, to obtain these beneficial attributes." (Greenwalt, et al, 1998). The bacteria and yeast are a balance of lactobacillus and Saccharomyces (including Saccharomyces boulardii). The Saccharomyces family is known to kill candida and pathogenic bacteria such as clostridia. It does NOT feed yeast. There have been rumors that yeast will promote candida growth. This is not true across the board. It depends on the type of yeast because some beneficial yeast kill pathogenic yeasts. People who have "sensitivities" and IgG reactions to yeasts such as baker's and brewer's yeast may have trouble with kombucha. I still believe this sensitivity may have started from an overgrowth of yeast or environmental mold and that ultimately these substances could help, but probably not at first. Another possible problem for some would be that as kombucha is made with black or green tea, both high in phenols, there may be some reaction to this part of the drink. Distinguishing between phenol reaction and yeast die-off may be a bit difficult but it is important. A "negative" reaction could simply be from killing the yeast. In my practice I have found that even those people with a sensitive to phenols can tolerate kombucha if they take No Fenol enzyme. As with all substances, start slowly.

One more thing on kombucha and fermented foods in general. They tend to be high in amines and for those with amine sensitivities, they may be problematic. See Appendix XIII for more information on foods high in amines and how to test for possible amine sensitivity.

If you look up the uses of kombucha online you will see a list that includes supporting digestion, metabolism, and immune system; weight and appetite control; improving liver function and alkalinity; anti-aging; cell integrity; and healthy skin and hair. Based on new and old research (this drink was very popular in the "old days" and much research was done in the 1920s through the 1960s, but there is also a significant amount of new research), some of the known active components in kombucha are:

- **Lactic Acid:** Found in Kombucha in its most potent form L-lactic(+). Lactic acid is essential for the digestive system.

- **Acetic Acid:** Its main function is to inhibit harmful bacteria. Acetic acid also conjugates toxins to neutralize them.

- **Malic Acid:** Is used in the body's detoxification process.

- **Oxalic Acid:** Encourages the cellular production of energy and is a natural preservative.

- **Glucuronic acid:** Is effective against many yeast infections such as candidiasis and thrush. Glucuronic acid is a wonderful detoxifier made by the liver to detoxify substances including petroleum-based products—one of the few agents capable of this. Once bound by glucuronic acid this substance is neutralized, cannot be reabsorbed, and is eliminated from the system.

- **Butyric Acid:** protects human cell membranes and combined with glucuronic acid strengthens the walls of the gut and protects against parasites and candida. Can also help with constipation.

- **Nucleic Acids:** Work with the body aiding healthy cell regeneration.

- **Amino Acids:** Amino acids have many benefits including building cells and repairing tissue. They also form antibodies to combat invading bacteria & viruses. L-theanine is one of the amino acids a client of mine calls the "yoga amino acid" as it has a calming effect on her (as it does most people) as though she just came from a yoga retreat.

- **Enzymes:** boost the actions of other health giving components

Kombucha also contains ascorbic acid (vitamin C), B vitamins (B1, B2, B3, B6, B12 and folic acid), beneficial yeasts and bacteria. Vitamin C and B-vitamins have many functions in the body and assist many systems including immune function.

Kombucha can be purchased at the store or made at home. I warn you ahead of time (jokingly), this beverage is delicious and may lead to an expensive habit if you buy it at the store. However, you can ferment it at home very inexpensively. It tastes nothing like black tea: it tastes like fermented apple cider, and people often add a bit of juice added for a variety of great flavors. Some favorite additions are gingerale, mango juice, guava juice, and many others. Although kombucha is made with sugar, the yeast and bacteria consume the sugar and what is left is about two grams of sugar in an eight ounce serving of kombucha.

Although there are different practitioners promoting different cultured foods, there is not a great deal of talk in the autism circles around using kombucha. I have been using it in my practice and have had positive feedback. Most kids love the taste too. I welcome feedback on your results and experience with kombucha. Please feel free to email me with your experience.

My website: www.HealthfulLiving.org contains a robust section of parent submitted recipes organized by diet, including GFCF, SCD, BED, special food sensitivities, grocery shopping lists, as well as instructions on how to make kombucha. You can find a kombucha culture online (such as the www.happyherbalist.com and others) or often a member of a Weston A. Price Foundation chapter near you.

#8 Refining the ASD Diet

By this point, most people have:
- Cleaned up the diet by eliminating artificial ingredients.
- Implemented a foundational ASD diet and done a three month (or so) trial.
- Removed any food sensitivities and other food intolerances.
- Started adding healthy nutrition boosters at the child's pace (this is an ongoing process).

Stop and celebrate! You have come a long way. Take a moment and look through old diet records to see what symptoms and behaviors have gone away or diminished. Stop and appreciate how far you and your child have come.

Now that you have gathered your thoughts on what you have accomplished, identify which symptoms still remain. Based on what you'd like to address next, go back and reread the ASD diet options and see what might apply best. This is the part of the process where people often start refining and layering diets—one on top of the other. They pick and chose additional principles to add or subtract from the current diet. Don't be afraid to experiment. Even if a food doesn't agree with someone it rarely will create a huge long-lasting regression—it's short lived and worth experimenting (once things are stable). After working with diet for a couple years, most children end up most successful with several dietary principles layered together. Here are some of the more common diets and substances to consider now:

- **Yeast/Body Ecology** – for yeast overgrowth, yeast symptoms, strong gas, digestive discomfort, and others. If you started with GFCF and you believe your child has yeast, you may want to implement a yeast diet, by either "adding" no sugars and moldy/yeasty foods to the GFCF diet, or "upgrading" the GFCF diet to the Body Ecology Diet. If you are on WAP or SCD, they already have some yeast principles—WAP with fermented foods and SCD for dysbiosis and gut inflammation—however, you may find applying more yeast principles helpful.

- **SCD** – for bowel inflammation, diarrhea, gut dysbiosis that is not improving. This diet is often the next step for those on GFCF with digestive issues that are not clearing up. Many people move to SCD and stay GFCF (i.e. not adding the yogurt, cheese, and butter). Others choose to stop GFCF and begin SCD. If the soaked or alkalizing grains of WAP and BED don't work, some will go to SCD or no grain diet (i.e. Paleo, GAPS).

- **Oxalates and the Low Oxalate Diet** – for pain (body, urinary, or GI), continued stimming, urinary incontinence or "playing with self," constipation or diarrhea. Often layered on top of SCD so someone would be doing the subset of foods allowed on SCD and LOD. While that is a common progression, some people just try removing high oxalate foods from whatever diet they are doing. In other cases, parents prefer to try soaking and fermenting grains, nuts, and beans first, instead of eliminating them.

- **Amines and the Failsafe** – Failsafe and amines take the Feingold diet a step further. If you discover that your child is sensitive to amines, and if rashes, headaches and pain, fatigue, and digestive problems persist, consider removing amines. Amines occur in many fermented foods. While these fermented foods are so helpful, if your child seems to be responding negatively to fermented or aged foods and you've ruled out yeast die-off, try Failsafe. See Appendix XI for a full list of salicylates, and Appendix XIII for a list of amines and free glutamate.

- **Lectins and GAPS/Paleo or soaking/fermenting** – Many of the diets that are helpful for the gut and candida address grains and their inflammatory effects. Some diets such as GAPS, SCD and Paleolithic diet remove these offenders. Other diets such as NT/WAP address these substances by breaking them down through soaking and fermentation. If gut issues or dysbiosis persist consider removing lectins or one of these diets that addresses them.

Choosing a diet and evolving a diet is an ongoing process for most. However, what about abandoning a diet altogether. There are times when progress is lost, even with strict adherence to a diet. The first thing to consider is whether it is a "positive regression," for example the opiate withdrawal from removing gluten. The second thing to consider is whether there could be any infractions in the diet. Next is whether there were any new additions or substitutions that caused a problem, for example amines from fermented foods. If it does not appear to be any of these areas, it is possible that some foundational components of biochemistry need to be addressed such as the need for antioxidants (vitamins A, C and E) or methyl B12. When methylation and other biochemical cascades are "stuck" or not working properly, possibly because key foundational nutrients are missing, it can be helpful to abandon a diet—go back to nourishing principles such as good quality fats, reduce grains or consume fermented grains, and getting as many nutrients in as possible. I know it is sometimes tempting to keep removing more and more foods as we assume they must be the problem since we are seeing some reaction. However, many times I find it valuable to go back to a less restrictive diet and work on some basic nutrient deficiencies and foundational digestive principles and preparations.

When refining the diet it's common for parents to want to make it stricter and stricter—as they see "reactions" it is easy to assume they must be food reactions, and they limit food choices more and more. There becomes this fear to add anything because their child seems to react to almost everything. And sometimes this is necessary. However, sometimes it's best to *expand* the diet. If it's too restrictive, there can be important nutrients missing.

#9 Cleaning up the Gut

Diets used to reduce yeast and dysbiosis (microbial imbalance) are listed above. In addition to diet, the following are a list of suggestions and substances frequently used to aid in cleaning up the gut. Supplements and protocols vary greatly between children depending on the types and resistance of certain gut bugs and bioindividuality. Many people choose to do a few of these suggestions or implement a yeast diet earlier on in the process—again that's very individual.

Balance Intestinal Flora and Support Digestion

In the days of our ancestors, fermented foods were essential to life. Fermentation allowed people to preserve vegetables for vitamins and nutrients in the winter, to prevent foods from spoiling, and for digestion and assimilation. In earlier times, we ate small amounts of fermented foods daily. Good bacteria help create a healthy environment to further the growth of other good bacteria and inhibit the growth of yeast and other pathogenic organisms.

Eat fermented foods (lactobaccilus fermentations such as yogurt and kefir, raw sauerkraut, and kombucha) liberally. I think fermented foods are one of the most important parts of a healthy diet for (almost) everyone. See my website for more information on fermented foods—what they are and how to prepare them.

With that said, I understand probiotic foods are "weird" and very sour, so some children won't eat them. A high quality probiotic supplement is important, especially for those who will not eat fermented foods. Quality varies greatly so it is important to get a professional line or something with multiple strains of lactobacillus and bifidobacterium with at least 10 billion bacteria per serving. See probiotics in *Impact of Nutrients*.

Eat a diet rich in fiber and low in refined carbohydrate (and starchy carbohydrate) to support flora growth. Of course, where these recommendation conflict with the current diet (i.e. SCD), do not implement them. Some simple guidelines to follow for feeding the good bacteria and balancing the internal terrain:
- Leafy greens.
- Root vegetables.
- Beans.
- Most green vegetables.
- Cruciferous family (unless cause digestive discomfort or problems with too much sulfur)
- One to two tablespoons of fresh ground flax seed daily.
- Limited grains (starchy), potatoes, corn.
- Avoid/eliminate sugar.
- Daily fermented foods.

Alkalizing the intestinal tract is a good way to make the environment healthy for good bacteria and inhospitable for yeast and other pathogens. Consuming any of these helps alkalize the system:
- Juice from one lemon/day
- 1 T apple cider vinegar/day

- Electrolytes
- Kombucha
- Bicarbonates are also important to assisting with the right pH in the small intestine for digestion and assimilation. The vitamin K Yahoo group at: http://health.groups.yahoo.com/group/VitaminK has some good information on bicarbonates.

Yeast (Candida)

For candida overgrowth, follow one of the several anti-yeast diets described above (for a basic one see Appendix IV) for a minimum of three months but preferably six months or more. Some people find they need to remain conscious of avoiding yeast-promoting foods for years. Continue to consume fermented foods and/or probiotics.

Yeast can become resistant to medications and supplements, so addressing yeast should be done with a strategy in mind. Often people choose several supplements that work on killing yeast in different ways to attack them from multiple angles. Parents often choose a few and stick with them for several months:

- **Start with probiotics:** Probiotics have properties that (while they don't kill yeast they) create an environment that does not allow yeast to thrive, weakening and crowding the yeast out. Probiotics are a key part of the process. However, this alone will not eradicate a significant yeast overgrowth.

- **Yeast to kill yeast:** Saccharomyces boulardii is a benign yeast that colonizes and then kills candida. Soon after you stop supplementing with it, it will leave the system. (Pangborn and Baker, 2002:183). However, as it is a yeast, those who are yeast *sensitive* (a yeast allergy) may not tolerate it. Kombucha is a fermented drink with saccharomyces boulardii that is often a wonderful addition.

- **Herbs with yeast killing properties:** Grapefruit seed extract, garlic, oregano oil, Oregon grape root, Indian fire tree bark. These are sold individually or in formulas.

- **Coconut:** Caprylic acid is a fatty acid found in coconut that kills yeast, as well as bacteria and viruses. Lauric acid is another fatty acid from coconuts that also has yeast, viral, and bacterial killing properties. Lauricidin or Monolaurin are two commercial products with lauric acid. Lauricidin is easier for children as it is small pellets that are easier than capsules—these are most often used for their anti-viral benefits. (Do note that anything that can attack viruses (Lauricidin, oregano oil) can actually cause more yeast in many ASD children. This does not mean these products are ineffective against yeast, but for some reason ASD children often become very yeasty during viral protocols, even unintentional ones.) Eating raw coconut oil and coconut milk are wonderful foods to add to the diet.

- **Enzymes** that include protease and cellulase help breakdown the cell walls of the yeast to weaken or kill them. Typically the enzymes are taken on an empty stomach; however, go with the label instructions. Candex by Pure Essence Labs is an enzyme product for yeast. See www.pureessencelabs.com

- **Transfer factors** with yeast specific antigens: Advanced Medical Labs has one called Transfer Factor 7000 at www.advancedmedicallabs.com.

- **Vitamins and minerals**: Biotin is helpful to keep yeast from being converted to a fungal state. Nutrients such as vitamin C and selenium that support the immune system are helpful.

- **Prescription antifungals**: Nystatin and Diflucan are prescription anti-fungals. While I cannot give advice on prescription medications, I can tell you that for some people they are very helpful; however, many DAN! doctors do not use them as a first line of attack for concern of creating resistant yeast.

- **Formulas**: There are many candida formulas out there such as Yeast-Aid by Kirkman that has a blend of anti-fungals and substances to fight yeast.

Just with multivitamin formulas, your child may be reactive to an ingredient in an anti-candida blend and may do better if you create your own blend of yeast supplements. Often parents choose: probiotics, enzymes, and a good diet to start. Remember diet is crucial. If you are feeding yeast with diet, the yeast killers will not work effectively.

While sulfur-rich supplements can be helpful for many conditions, they can feed yeast. If you are dealing with a big yeast problem, you may need to avoid supplements such as taurine, alpha lipoic acid, DMSA, NAC, and glutathione. Do note however, that for many people chelation has proved key to finally getting yeast under control, and both alpha lipoic acid and DMSA are effective chelation agents.

As candida dies it gives off toxins and gas. To neutralize these effects try either activated charcoal or Alka Seltzer Gold. Activated charcoal absorbs toxins in the gut including toxins given off during yeast die off. Typically dosing is four to eight capsules per day according to Pangborn and Baker (Pangborn and Baker, 2001) one-half to two capsules, two to three times per day according to Bock (Bock, 2007). Take activated charcoal away from medications, supplements and food, as it will absorb these compounds as well. For Alka Seltzer Gold, dose according to label—be sure it is Gold, as this Alka Seltzer product is strictly bicarbonate.

Parasites

Of course, you'll want to eliminate any parasites and pathogenic organisms. A stool test can help identify parasites; although, parasites can be elusive and difficult to find. (see assessment in the Impact of Nutrients section). The following natural anti-parasitic remedies can often kill parasites. Work with a physician while trying to rid parasites, as testing and medication may be necessary. Parasite remedies include:

- Medicinal mushrooms – Certain medicinal mushrooms kill parasites. Host Defense by New Chapter and Myco-Immune by Thorne are two medicinal mushroom blends.
- Citrus seed.
- Clove.
- Black walnut and wormwood.

- Paracide by Wise Woman Herbals (wisewomanherbals.com) is one of many herbal parasite formulas. The taste is quite strong.
- Soil based probiotics (Garden of Life's Primal Defense) appear to have anti-parasite properties as well.
- Homeopathy is often quite helpful.
- Additionally, there are machines (through sound, vibration, and other means) that generate frequencies that kill harmful microorganisms that you can access through a qualified professional.
- Prescription medication may be a good option if natural remedies are not effective. Ask your physician to prescribe a pharmaceutical.

Supplements to Help the Gut

As you remove yeast and other pathogenic organisms from the gut, you can choose to use supplements that have proven helpful to gut healing.

- Aloe juice—one tablespoon, up to three times daily (can cause diarrhea if too much) (Zand, 1994:314). Aloe is a mucilaginous polysaccharide that is soothing and allows the gut to repair itself. However, on SCD these polysaccharides can feed dysbiosis can create a gut problem. There is nothing inherently wrong with aloe, only with polysaccharide sensitive people. George's Aloe removes the inflammatory substances that are just under the rind that irritate the digestive tract, so it's a good brand to try, especially as it has no taste.
- Slippery Elm—(1/2 tsp in six oz water daily) (Tilgner, 1999:108 and Zand, 1994:23).
- Marshmallow—as tea (Zand, 1994:22)
- BrainChild Nutritionals' IntestiMend product.
- Butyrate (or butyric acid)—nourishes the intestinal lining and contains antimicrobial properties. Butyric acid is found in raw butter and dairy products. For those not consuming dairy, butyric acid is available is casein-free supplement form.
- Vitamin A—cod liver oil contains vitamin A, which aids tissue repair and helps heal leaky gut. (Thurnham, 2000).

While glutamine is helpful for healing the gut, it is neuro-excitatory for some (causing hyperactivity) and may even "over excite" neurons to death for some with glutamate sensitivity or "leaky blood brain barrier" (insufficient sulfation with GAGs or open calcium gates allowing brain cells to continually fire). Although great for the average adult, I don't usually recommend glutamine for children on the autistic spectrum. Additionally, many of the mucilaginous fibers (aloe, slippery elm) are not allowed on SCD.

Probiotics and fermented foods also help heal the gut. Nutrient dense foods provide more nutrients to aid with healing as well.

#10 Supplement Specifics

Once you have had a chance to clean up the diet and determine what to eat, you will begin to see certain symptoms clear up. With that, you'll also see what symptoms still remain. From here, you can determine what supplements to add next. These may include more specific nutrients for improving methylation/sulfation, nutrients to boost immune function, heal the gut, and/or reduce inflammation. See the sections *Importance of Nutrients* and *Nutrient Protocol for Autism* for more details of supplements that are often helpful.

- Inositol
- NAC/Glutathione
- Sulfates
- Amino acids
- DMAE

- Colostrum
- Butyric acid
- Medicinal mushrooms
- Transfer factors
- NAG/Glyconutrients

- Biotin
- Vitamin D
- Vitamin K
- Herbs

Continue adding supplements one at a time as needed. If you notice a regression, assess what might be causing it and adjust as necessary. For example, is the child feeding yeast with NAC, or unable to process an amino acid? If so, back up and slow down, or switch to another form or formula, or discontinue altogether.

#11 Support Immune Function

There are two important areas of the immune support relating to autism. The first is having the anti-viral and anti-fungal defenses to fight off pathogenic organisms. The second is regulating inflammation and the anti-inflammatory response.

Viral/Bacterial Defense

Th1 (T-helper 1) and Th2 (T-helper 2) arms of the immune system need to be in balance. As we mentioned earlier, Th1 is often low with Th2 predominating. A number of supplements can help regain the balance between the two arms of the immune system. Omega-3 fatty acids of both EPA and DHA and Omega-9 (oleic acid in olive oil) are very beneficial to Th1 lymphocytes. Vitamin A (in the natural cis form) is also very important for immune function and Th1 activity. Vitamin C increases Th1 while suppressing Th2. Vitamins E and B complex can increase Th1. Both panax ginseng and glyconutrients can also increase Th1. "Raising glutathione levels has been shown to alter the cytokine balance in favor of a Th1 immune response" (Peterson, 1998) and can be done by adding NAC or milk thistle (although Dr. John Hicks does not recommend milk thistle for children). Vitamin C and E, selenium, and all antioxidants spare glutathione. For more ways to boost glutathione see step #12 Detoxification.

Probiotics provide an enormous set of functions for us including supporting the immune system and increasing the number of immune cells. Nutrients such as zinc, selenium, vitamin C, E, B6, and the amino acids glutamine, cysteine, and arginine are important for immune function. Carotenes (such as beta carotene for one) enhance immune response and allow glutathione to be saved for detoxification functions.

Both colostrum and transfer factor are good support for the immune system and to fight off pathogens. Transfer factors are much more concentrated as compared to colostrum. Transfer factors are antigen specific and there are particular transfer factors to fight various microbes such as candida. Medicinal mushrooms such as reishi, shiitake, and maitake have powerful immune system benefits including killing yeast, bacteria, and viruses as well as boosting natural killer cells. EpiCor is a yeast-based product that stimulates and nourishing the immune system.

Supporting the endocrine system including the adrenals and thyroid is important to supporting the immune system. When stress is high, cortisol, a hormone produced by the adrenals, increases and DHEA, another hormone, decreases. DHEA assists Th1 function. An adrenal or hormone panel can tell you if cortisol is high and/or DHEA is low. When needed, it is helpful to support the adrenals with adrenal glandulars or adaptagenic herbs (see *Impact of Nutrients*)—supporting the adrenals helps to avoid excess cortisol and help balance the organ.

Reducing Inflammation

Reducing inflammation can be done by avoiding inflammatory foods and substances, and increasing the amount of anti-inflammatory foods, herbs/spices, and supplements. Inflammatory foods include any food sensitivities and naturally inflammatory foods (such as acid-forming foods). The following are anti-inflammatory foods to focus on and inflammatory foods to avoid.

Anti-inflammatory	Inflammatory
• Pomegranate • Berries • Goji berries • Apple • Hemp seeds • Almonds, walnuts and most nuts/seeds • Coconut oil/coconut milk/coconut butter • Cucumber • Shiitake mushrooms • Broccoli and cruciferous vegetables • Squash • Celery • Potatoes and sweet potatoes • Green vegetables rich in chlorophyll • Fish oil • Fennel • Burdock • Chamomile • Fenugreek • Flax seed • Ginger • Licorice • Plantain • Slippery elm • Spirulina • Turmeric • Wheat grass • Yucca • Pycnogenol	• Sugar • Maple sugar/syrup • White flour • High fructose corn syrup • Corn syrup • Trans fats • Margarine • Commercial grain-fed meat • Commercial cold cereal • Non-soaked and -fermented wheat (commercially prepared) • Soy • Corn • Deep fried foods • Soda • Cookies and other desserts • Artificial sweeteners • Eggplant and other nightshades • Oxalates • Non-soaked and -fermented grains (rice, oats, rye, quinoa, millet)

#12 Detoxification

There are many ways to support detoxification. One of the first steps (after avoiding toxins) is supporting the organs of detoxification. In the supplement section, *Impact of Nutrients*, there is a list of herbs that support the liver, kidneys, and the detoxification pathways. Chelation is a specific method of heavy metal detoxification that chelates (or binds to) metals such as mercury and lead. There are other forms of heavy metal detoxification that are not chelation. Physical detoxification such as sweating, baths, and saunas are another great way to support detoxification—through the skin.

Supporting Detoxification

Regarding detoxification pathways, the liver has two main phases—I and II. Often we need to boost phase II in autism. Here are various ways to support detoxification and phases I and II specifically:

1) **Reduce toxic exposure**: Decrease exposure to phenolic compounds, environmental toxins, heavy metals and anything that would tax an overburdened system. Tylenol wipes out the entire supply of PST within minutes and should be avoided scrupulously. Additionally, Prozac and Diflucan are fluoride-containing medications, which load the body with fluoride. Remember, never stop or change a medication without supervision of a physician—my point is to be aware of everything that might be influencing toxic exposure and then proceed accordingly. The following are substances to stay away from that overburden Phase I: benzene such as gasoline, 1,4-diclororbenzede such as mothballs and room deodorizers, sylene in deodorants, room fresheners, paint vapors, dioxin in herbicides, auto exhaust, styrene in Styrofoam, ketones, and aldehydes (formaldehyde and candida toxins). As well, I would assume phthalates/plastics and most toxins would burden Phase 1.

2) **Increase Phase II detoxification**: Glutathione conjugation is enhanced by cruciferous vegetables such as cabbage, broccoli, brussels sprouts, amino acid conjugation by glycine, methylation by lipotropic nutrients such as choline, methionine, betaine, folic acid, and B12, and sulfation by cysteine, methionine and taurine. L-Glycine is an amino acid (that along with cysteine and glutamine makes glutathione). Glycine is also the main ingredient for the Phase II detoxification pathway that clears phenols, salicylates, benzoates, and excess organic acids. Methionine, betaine, and choline enhance liver function and increase the levels of SAM and glutathione. In addition to the above supplements, enhancing glutathione is important, especially as it is low in most with ASD. Vitamin A, C, and E, zinc, selenium, and carotenes enhance immune response and "spare" glutathione. Milk thistle increases Phase II by assisting glutathione-S-transferase (GST), a Phase II enzyme that adds a glutathione group to Phase I products. Milk thistle increases glutathione production up to 35%, but does not directly stimulate the enzyme.

3) **Increase Phase I function**: Magnesium, zinc, vitamin C, vitamins B2, B3, B6, and B12, and folic acid are needed by phase I detoxification. Antioxidants such as milk thistle, pregnenolone, phosphatidylcholine, and turmeric support Phase I. Milk thistle increases both Phase I and II. Milk thistle (and its active ingredient silymarin) is also a potent liver protector and regenerator. However, milk thistle can be counterproductive or dangerous when PST (Phase II) is low as it increases Phase I to a greater degree than Phase II.

4) **Decrease Phase I function**: Many substances that people see benefit from may be in part due to their ability to slow down Phase I. As I mentioned, we wouldn't normally want to slow down Phase I but some people do see great improvements with these substances and that may be because it is slowing down the flood of toxic metabolites to an overburdened Phase II. Therefore, if Phase II is very slow, decreasing Phase I can be helpful so substances such as phenols don't build up to dangerous amounts as in those with faulty PST and phenol sensitivity. Substances which can slow down Phase I function include: grapefruit seed extract (Citricidal ™), naringenin from grapefruit juice, strawberries, raspberries, Diflucan and possibly other antifungals (according to Schauss). There are probably more of these substances but the desire it to increase Phase 2 so there is no "bottleneck" of toxins. I suppose the more important point is if you see a

positive reaction to *long term* use of anti-fungals that regresses everytime the medication is stopped, Schauss suggests people suspect this downregulation effect is creating the benefit (more than killing yeast).

As we have discussed, most of those with ASD have toxic burdens and/or detoxification insufficiencies. We know that mercury causes serious brain, cellular, and biochemical damage and disruption. It is one of the most toxic substances our children can be exposed to, especially the ethylmercury form found in thimerosal. There are even those who feel that the correct diagnosis for some is not autism but actually mercury toxicity. I know from my own personal experience that upon receiving test results which show high mercury levels our first reaction is "Remove it! And remove it as fast as possible!" There is some accuracy to that feeling because there are many who feel that the younger the child is when the metal is removed, the less damage has occurred and the sooner and more thoroughly the child can recover.

While the toxicity of mercury is evident, and the need to detoxify it is great, I feel we should be cautious in our approach to detoxification. It's important to get the mercury (and other metals) out; however, it can be very harmful to do so the wrong way. The first place to start is to find a good doctor to remove it. Do not assume just because someone is a "DAN! doctor" he or she is experienced with chelation. Ask other parents. Talk to the physicians and find out their approach.

Chelation

There is little doubt that a great many ASD children have had their health damaged by toxic metals, including mercury, lead, aluminum, cadmium, antimony, arsenic, and others. Many parents have found that the most effective way to remove these toxic metals, and improve health, is through a process called chelation. At 73%, chelation has the highest rating as a treatment for ASD children (Autism Research Institute Parent Ratings).

To remove the metals, a chelating agent is introduced to the body. The chemical composition of the agent allows it to bind to sequestered metals, pulling them from where they have settled. There is a second, equally important phase to chelation, and that is allowing the body enough time and support to ensure that the metal now bound to the chelating agent is safely excreted.

Generally, most ASD children are being chelated with one or more of the following agents: DMSA, DMPS, ALA, and EDTA. There is much controversy regarding chelation, even among practitioners who treat ASD biomedically. Controversy includes how best to introduce the chelating agent (orally, transdermally, intravenously, or as a suppository), how often to dose, how much to dose, how to choose the best chelator for the situation, how to measure success, how to know when you are finished, how to support the body during chelation, and what side effects are acceptable. As with all biomedical interventions, it is important that parents research and make decisions for their child. This may be especially important for chelation, as compared to, for example, introducing a new supplement, because there are higher risks associated with chelation if it is done improperly.

DAN! practitioners seem to practice many protocols for chelation. Many of the recent approaches to DAN! chelation techniques can be found here, at the ARI website: http://www.autism.com/treatable/index.htm#chelation. Because of the many approaches to chelation used by DAN! practitioners (and non-DAN! practitioners as well) it is important to verify which approach yours is recommending. Many DAN! doctors are now using IV and suppository chelation, as well as oral and transdermal, although far fewer are using transdermal chelation now. Transdermal chelators were very popular until recently, when it was discovered that they are quite ineffective in pulling metals for most children. Many parents are seeing success with IV and suppository chelation; however, it cannot be ignored that there are parent reports of regression on these more aggressive forms of chelation. As with any intervention, it makes sense to investigate the proven therapies that are the least invasive and most proven in terms of safety and efficacy. Parents must then take this information and apply it to the unique situation of their own child.

A very important point to consider when chelating is how the chelating agents work in the body. Andrew Hall Cutler, Ph.D., a chemist, has based his protocol on the half-life of chelating agents (that is, how long it takes for half of the chelator to clear the blood), and argues that it is very important to keep a relatively steady level of the chelator in the blood because the chelators we have available to us now are known to drop the metals they have picked up (that is, a metal will be picked up and dropped many times by the chelating agent before it is excreted). Cutler argues that if we do not take half-life and the inability of chelators to hang on to metals permanently into consideration, the metals can be redistributed to other parts of the body rather than safely excreted. Cutler also argues that supporting the body with proper supplements is crucial to ensuring safe and comfortable chelation. Cutler's protocol and other information can be found at http://groups.yahoo.com/group/Autism-Mercury. He has also written two helpful books you can find in the resource section.

Dr. Amy Yasko takes a much different view of chelation than either Cutler or DAN!. Her approach has been used on far fewer children; however, one may find her ideas here http://www.ch3nutrigenomics.com/phpBB2/welcome.html.

In researching, especially on the internet, a parent will find many claims of "safe" and "natural" chelators. It does appear that some of these products seem to result in some benefit for a percentage of ASD children. However, it would be wrong to assume that just because something is touted as "natural" that it is effective, or even safe. Alpha lipoic acid, the preferred chelator of Dr. Cutler for many reasons, including the fact that it can cross the blood brain barrier and remove metals from the brain, is a natural product that provides many substantial benefits to the body; however, if used improperly, it can actually worsen symptoms of mercury poisoning. (Rooney, 2007) As another example, some people prefer not to use DMSA because it is a synthetic drug; however, in his latest research, Dr. James Adams has discovered that glutathione levels, both low and high, were normalized in ASD children after just one round of chelation with oral DMSA (publication pending).

Chelation has proven a very successful intervention for hundreds of ASD children; however, it is worth repeating that because chelation, particularly certain methods of chelation, may pose a higher risk than other interventions, a parent should gather as much information from as many sources as possible before making decisions as to how to approach this treatment.

Sweating and Far Infrared Sauna

Another way to detoxify that uses a completely different method of detox from the ones discussed above is the far infrared sauna. There is much evidence on sweating in general to remove not only heavy metals but other toxins as well. Additionally, far infrared technology, which has been studied extensively in Japan, is an even more effective way than sweating alone. The benefit to this is that using the skin as a primary detoxification route; it bypasses the gut, liver, and kidneys, which are often not in the best condition to detoxify. As the toxins come out through the skin, the internal organs are not as affected and it creates little body burden on the organs, as compared to normal chelation. Additionally, research shows that detoxification with far infrared sauna helps eliminate other environmental toxins such as PCBs as well. Be aware, many people who are toxic do not sweat. In these cases, you need to go very slowly when introducing the far infrared sauna. Additionally, sweating will deplete nutritive minerals to some extent so supplementation is important.

I have a far infrared sauna in my practice and use it personally. I love using it as I always feel great, cleansed and refreshed after I finish. It is not like traditional saunas that can make you feel depleted and wiped out after use. The far infrared sauna is a great detoxification program for the whole family. Many of my clients own them and are finding them helpful.

There are many saunas on the market. Two of the major ones are Heavenly Heat Saunas and High Tech Health. High Tech Health's website has a wonderful list of research papers on the use of far infrared saunas (not brand specific) and sweating for detoxification at www.hightechhealth.com/sauna_pdfs/references_sauna.pdf. The marketing information can get confusing but two important points are to get a sauna without any glue and without cedarwood (contain aromatic oils many are sensitive to).

Progress and Regression

Charting progress is an important step along the way. Documentation is often essential in order to determine what any reactions may be due to. It's important to record the diet with supplements, any dietary or supplement changes, and any physical, emotional, cognitive, digestive, and bowel changes you see. It is hard to remember back, especially with so many things going on.

To reiterate, you may not need to do all of the steps I have outlined. You also may need to address some steps more than once. Therefore, do not be overwhelmed by the steps or their order. The idea is to give you a place to start and an idea of what general order to address things.

There are regressions that will happen along the way. Your child many suddenly get irritable, hyperactive, or bowel movements may change. This is common. When you change anything, something is going to result. Your job is to determine whether it is what one of my clients calls a "positive" or "negative" regression. I describe a positive regression as short-term healing symptoms. An example is irritability caused by opiate withdrawal from removing gluten. A "negative" regression is a sign that the change cannot be tolerated by the individual, for example, hyperactivity from B6 or diarrhea from corn when wheat was replaced.

This can cause understandable frustration for the individual or parent, when everything is going well and then suddenly some of the gains are lost or symptoms such as diarrhea appear. If a new symptom appears or reemerges after a supplement is added, go back to the original schedule for a day or two, and slowly increase. If symptoms continue, ask a physician or professional for their advice. If a diet causes regression, notice what foods were increased and consider any reactions to them. Confirm you are doing the diet correctly—one infraction can cause problems sometimes. If the diet or supplement is not working, try another approach—another form of the nutrient, even another diet.

The following are examples of a diet record and supplement chart, for ways to track progress. Everyone has their own way, and I can't stress enough the value of a diet record and/or progress chart. There are electronic copies available on my website that you can modify for your own use. NourishingHope.com.

Daily Food / Mood Record

1. *Please write out you child's daily diet. Fill out a diet record for at least two days. Include portion size and any supplements or medications.   Include time of day.*
2. *Additionally, record any symptoms you feel during or after eating, such as drowsy, irritable, energized.*

	Time	Food/Supplements	Mood/Energy/Symptoms
Example	9:00am	*1 cups of Cheerios with ¾ c cow milk* *1 multi-vitamin, 500 mg vit C*	*10:00 Feel fine* *11:00 Low energy, stressed*
Breakfast			
Snack			
Lunch			
Snack			
Dinner			
Night-time			

Daily Supplement Schedule

	Supplement	Notes
Early Morning		
Breakfast		
Mid morning		
Lunch		
Afternoon		
Dinner		
Bedtime		

As this book is not intended as medical advice, any times symptoms persist or you feel something is wrong, ask a physician for help. A nutritionist can help with dietary implementation and determining an approach. Seek assistance from other parents or a professional. Parents are some of the most educated people I know and their experience is invaluable.

Ultimately, the parents are in charge of the course of intervention. Seek a team of support but be educated and aware enough of the biochemistry, symptoms and conditions so you can guide the care and support you receive. Keeping a record of progress will really help you and your team piece together what to try next.

CONCLUSION

The purpose of this book is to empower parents, families, practitioners, and those with autism. We now know that autism is not strictly a *psychological* disorder for which nothing can be done. It is a *neurological* disorder resulting from biochemical imbalances. These imbalances, which may be the result of genetic susceptibility and various environmental assaults, manifest in psychological and physical symptoms. Understanding and continuing to discover the biochemical processes that impact psychology, behavior, and social interaction among these individuals with autistic spectrum disorders, provide great hope and possibility for improvement for affected individuals. The more we know, the more we can discover new ways to offer support through nutrient supplementation and holistic intervention.

As I have illustrated, addressing the biochemistry and system/organ function can contribute to diminishing symptoms of autism, even leading to recovery. I have spoken with many families who've shared stories of how their child was on the autistic spectrum but after various therapies including nutrition and supplement intervention their child was re-diagnosed as *not* on the autistic spectrum. I'm not specifying one approach that works for all. Instead, I'm suggesting that by balancing the biochemistry and body systems children can get better—sometimes a little better, sometimes a full recovery.

I believe, for any being, the physical, psychological, emotional, and spiritual aspects must be in balance for optimal health. The next step on my journey is to better understand the spiritual and energetic impacts of autism. We, as holistic practitioners, understand that events, trauma, and thoughts are stored in the body on the cellular level. We are discovering on a daily basis that subtle energy has an impact on the physical and biochemical. Just ask anyone who has made themselves sick with worry. Asking the body for guidance on healing and clearing the stagnant energy can also be important steps to recovery. I am excited to explore these areas. I have more and more clients (including myself) who have explored subtle energy therapies (acupuncture, cranialsacral therapy, homeopathy, Bioset, and other energy work) and many tell me, "I don't know how it works but it made positive changes." A parent, Amy Lansky used homeopathy for her son to rid him of his autism diagnosis and wrote a wonderful book, *Impossible Cure: The Promise of Homeopathy*. While we may not know how it works yet, science is making new discoveries in quantum physics and other realms that measure the impact of energy. The section "Additional Author's Comments" goes into more detail on subtle energy.

I encourage people to have faith and persevere on their journeys of learning and healing, as what they uncover impacts so many lives. Nourish yourself and your family along your journey—it will help all of you. And remember, there is always hope.

APPENDICES

Appendix I - Developmental Characteristics of Autism

Social	Communication
No interest in friends	Difficulty with conversation
Does not imitate	Lacks imagination
Avoids eye contact	Does not use gestures ("bye-bye")
Not playful	Reverses pronouns ("you" and "I")
Prefers own company to being with others	Cannot communicate with words or gestures

Unusual Interests	Behavioral
Fascination with facts	Hand flapping
Lines toys in neat rows	Picky eating habits
Intensely interested in mechanical workings	"Stimming"
Reads words at a very early age, but does not use the words to communicate	Injures self or others
	Physically inactive or passive
	Throws frequent tantrums

Appendix Ia – Physical Characteristics of Autism

Physical		
Tics	Constipation	Difficulty sleeping
Headaches	Diarrhea	Asthma
Vomiting	Muscle aches	Ear infections
Hives	Fatigue	Bedwetting

Source: Powers, 2000:10-11 and various research

Appendix II - Comparison of Characteristics of Mercury Poisoning & Autism

Characteristic	Mercury Poisoning	Autism
Movement disorders	Arm flapping, ankle jerks, rocking, circling; uncoordinated, clumsiness; inability to walk, stand, or sit; difficulty swallowing or chewing; walking on the toes	Arm flapping, jumping, spinning, rocking, circling; abnormal posture and gait; clumsiness, uncoordinated; difficulties crawling, lying down, sitting, walking; difficulty swallowing or chewing; walking on the toes
Sensory abnormalities	Oversensitive to sound; abnormal sensation in the mouth, arms, and legs; doesn't like to be touched	Oversensitive to sound; abnormal sensation in the mouth, arms, and legs; doesn't like to be touched
Speech, hearing, language problems	Loss of speech or failure to develop speech; hearing loss; deafness at very high doses; problems with articulation; word retrieval problems	Delayed language or failure to develop speech; mild to severe hearing loss; problems with articulation; word use errors
Cognitive problems	Borderline intelligence, mental retardation: may be reversed; poor concentration and attention; difficulty following complex commands; difficulty comprehending words; difficulty understanding abstract ideas and symbols	Borderline intelligence, mental retardation: may be recovered; poor concentration, shifting attention; difficulty following multiple commands; difficulty comprehending words; difficulty understanding abstract ideas and symbols
Visual problems	Poor eye contact; blurred vision	Poor eye contact; blurred vision
Physical problems	Decreased muscle strength, especially in upper body, incontinence, salivating; rash, dermatitis; abnormal sweating, poor circulation, high heart rate; diarrhea, constipation, abdominal pain; anorexia, nausea, poor appetite; seizures; sensitive individuals more likely to have allergies, asthma; more likely to have autoimmune symptoms, especially rheumatoid	Decreased muscle strength, especially in upper body, incontinence; rash, dermatitis; abnormal sweating, poor circulation, high heart rate; diarrhea, constipation, gas, abdominal discomfort anorexia, feeding problems; seizures; tendency to have allergies and asthma; family history of autoimmune symptoms, especially rheumatoid arthritis
Unusual behavior	Sleeping difficulties; injures self, such as head banging; staring, unprovoked crying, social isolation	

Source: Cave, 2001:63-64. Original information adapted from "Autism: A Unique Type of Mercury Poisoning" by Sallie Bernard et al. rewritten in *What Your Doctor May Not Tell You About Children's Vaccinations* by Stephanie Cave.

Summary Comparison of Biological Abnormalities in Mercury Exposure and Autism

Mercury Exposure	Autism
Biochemistry	
Binds –SH groups; blocks sulfate transporter in intestines, kidneys	Low sulfate levels
Reduces glutathione availability; inhibits enzymes of glutathione metabolism; glutathione needed in neurons, cells and live to detoxify heavy metals; reduces glutathione peroxidase and reductase	Low levels of glutathione; decreased ability of liver to detoxify xenobiotics; abnormal glutathione peroxidase activity in erythrocytes
Disrupts purine and pyrimidine metabolism	Purine and pyrimidine metbolism errors lead to autistic feature
Disrupts mitochondrial activities, especially in brain	Mitochondrial dysfunction, especially in brain
Immune system	
Sensitive individuals more likely to have allergies, asthma, autoimmune-like symptoms, especially rheumatoid-like ones	More likely to have allergies and asthma; familial presence of autoimmune diseases, especially rheumatoid arthritis; IgA deficiencies
Can produce an immune response in CNS; causes brain/MBP autoantibodies	On-going immune response in CNS; brain/MBP autoantibodies present
Causes overproduction of Th1 subset; hills/inhibits lymphocytes, T-cells, and monocytes; decreases NKT-cell activity; induces or suppresses IFNg and IL-2	Skewed immune-cell subset in the Th2 direction; decreased responses to T-cell mitogens; reduces NK T-cell function; increased IFNg and IL-12
CNS structure	
Selectively targets brain areas unable to detoxify or reduce	Specific areas of brain pathology; many functions spared
Hg-induced oxidative stress	Pathway in amygdala, hippocampus, basal ganglia, cerebral cortex; damage to Purkinje and granulae cells in cerebellum; brain stem defects in some cases
Accumulates in amygdala, hippocampus, basal ganglia, cerebral cortex; damages Purkinje and granule cells in cerebellum; brain stem defects in some cases	Neuronal disorganization; increased neuronal cell replication, increased glial cells; depressed expression of NCAMs
Causes abnormal neuronal cytoarchitecture; disrupts neuronal migration, microtubules, and cell division; reduces NCAMs	Progressive microcephaly and macrocephaly
Progressive microcephaly	

Neuro-Chemistry	
Prevents presynaptic serotonin release and inhibits serotonin transport; causes calcium disruptions	Decreased serotonin synthesis in children; abnormal calcium metabolism
Alters dopamine systems; peroxidine deficiency in rates resembles mercurialism in humans	Either high or low dopamine levels; positive response to peroxidine, which lowers dopamine levels
Elevates epinephrine and norepinephrine levels by blocking enzyme that degrades epinephrine	Elevated norepinephrine and epinephrine
Elevates glutamate	Elevates gluamate and asparate
Leads to cortical ecetylcholine deficiency; increases muscarinic receptor density in hippocampus and cerebellum	Cortical acetaylchoine deficiency; reduced muscarinic receptor binding in hipporcampus
Causes demyelinating neuropathy	Demyelination in brain
Neurophysiology	
Causes abnormal EEGs, epileptiform activity, variable patterns, e.g. subtle, low amplitude seizure activities	Abnormal EEGs, epileptiform activity, variable patterns, including subtle low amplitude seizure activities
Causes abnormal vestibular nystagmus responses; loss of sense of position in space	Abnormal vestibular nystagmus responses; loss of sense of position in space
Results in autonomic disturbance; excessive sweating, poor circulation, elevated heart rate	"Autonomic disturbance; unusual sweating, poor circulation, elevated heart rate

Source: "Autism: a Novel Form of Mercury Poisoning" by Bernard et al, 2001, pg 465.

Appendix III - Points to Consider for Vaccination

As you have seen, there is evidence that vaccinations, either due to mercury (alone, or working synergistically with other metals) and/or the live viruses, may be one of the etiological events leading to autism. For this reason, parents should be well informed and take a cautious approach to vaccinations. I am not against vaccinations or suggesting that vaccinations not be given to children. Vaccinations are a personal decision; however, I am suggesting that you do your own research on vaccinations, weigh the pros and cons, and decide for yourself which vaccines you would like to give to your children (if any), in what combination, and at what age. Do not be pressured by other parents, the school, or the medical system to vaccinate your children. Most states, including California, allow for exemptions based on religious, medical or philosophical reasons. The following are guidelines to consider that I have compiled from Drs. Elizabeth Cave, Jon Pangborn, Sidney Baker, Gary Null and others, regarding vaccinations for children. This information is not intending as medical advice - it is educational only. Use this information to have a conversation with your physician, to do more research on the subject, and to consider all of the options.

- Avoid unnecessary combinations of vaccines (such as the MMR and DTaP). Currently, MMR is available in single shots where measles, mumps, and rubella can be given in separate shots at different doctor visits. However, DTaP is not been available separately.
- Space vaccinations by as much time as possible, ideally a minimum of six months.
- Research at what age you want to start vaccinations or give particular vaccinations. Certain systems such as the brain and nervous system are not fully formed or undergo significant growth until 2 years of age. Weigh the pros and cons of waiting.
- Use mercury free-vaccines (They are available for many vaccines but you need to call ahead so your doctor can order them. As they are more expensive, they are not automatically used. Also remember that they are not truly mercury-free, but are in fact just mercury reduced).
- Demand to see the package and label to ensure the proper mercury-free vaccine.
- Use single-dose vials from which to draw the vaccine because the dose is more uniform.
- Use inactivated polio (the shot, not the oral form).
- Do not vaccinate your child if he or she is sick or recovering from an illness or infection.
- Wait on vaccines if your child has been around or cared for by someone with an immune system disorder like cancer, AIDS, or leukemia.
- Hold off on vaccines if your child has had treatments that tax the immune system, such as x-rays, cortisone, or other steroid drugs.
- Get a copy of the Vaccine Information Statement from your physician before the next vaccine so you can have time to read about it. Also, do your own homework and study the risk of serious illness or death from the disease versus the risk of the vaccine (in causing autism or to damage to the immune system in general).
- Give a bigger than usual supplement of vitamin A (1250-5000 IU per day of cod liver oil) to your child three days before and the day of the shot. Also, give vitamin C for three days before the shot and the day of the shot—100 mg for infants and 300 mg for toddlers.
- Prioritize vaccines in order of greatest chance of exposure. For example, there is a much greater chance that school children might be exposed to hemophilus influenza type B(HiB) and polio,

both with can have serious effects on children, as opposed to hepatitis B which is transmitted through IV drug use, sexual intercourse, and when the mother has hepatitis B. Since the chance of an infant or child getting hepatitis B is very rare (except when the mother is infected and those tests are routinely performed), why would a child be given this vaccine? Even more alarming is the fact that it is recommended in the pediatric immunization schedule to be given at *birth* (within hours or days of life)!

- Have your child's level of antibodies checked instead of blindly giving the additional recommended boosters. For example, five DTaP shots are scheduled but all may not be necessary to reach adequate antibody levels. In fact, the majority of people have appropriate titers after one vaccination.
- Avoid re-immunization with a vaccine after a previous bad reaction by the child or a sibling.
- Do not immunize newborns.
- Mother should avoid vaccinations while pregnant and postpartum while breastfeeding.

Appendix IV - Yeast Diet

Eliminate all antibiotics, steroids, immune-suppressing drugs (with supervision of a physician)

Eliminate the following foods:
- All refined and simple sugars, including barley malt, artificial sweeteners, maple syrup, and chocolate. Instead, use stevia or xylitol.
- Eliminate milk and other dairy products.
- Foods high in yeast, mold, or fungus such as cheeses, dried fruits, melons, peanuts, mushrooms, corn and rye.
- Vinegar-ferments such as vinegar, soy sauce, Worcestershire sauce, pickles, vanilla extract.
- Fruit: Best to eliminate for the first three to four weeks. If not, at least eliminate apples and grapes (and all products made with them).
- Hot dogs, salami, processed lunchmeats.
- Baked goods containing yeast including bread.
- Eliminate all processed foods, and artificial flavors, colors, and preservatives.

What to eat:
- Chicken, turkey (unprocessed), beef, fish.
- Vegetables.
- Quinoa, amaranth, millet.
- Beans.
- Brown rice.
- Tomatoes.
- Herbs.
- Ghee or vegetable oil.
- Berries.
- Stevia or xylitol.
- Root vegetables such as sweet potatoes and parsnips.

Add one more of the following with guidance from a practitioner:
- Oregano oil.
- Garlic supplements.
- Oregon Grape Root.
- Grapefruit seed extract.
- Caprylic acid/MCT oil.
- Sacchromyces Boulardii.
- Probiotic: 25-100 billion CFUs of viable lactobacillus acidophilus, bactobacillus bifidum, and other probiotic strains.
- Klaire Labs: Ther-Biotic Complete, Ther-Biotic Detox (www.klairelabs.com).
- Kirkman Labs: Super Pro-Bio Gold (www.kirkmanlabs.com).
- Custom Probiotics brand is one of the few without SCD illegal fillers such as inulin (www.customprobiotics.com).

- ThreeLac: Helpful for yeast overgrowth (www.globalhealthtrax.com).
- VSL3: contains 450 Billion bacteria (www.vsl3.com).
- Primal Defense: start with 1/2 scoop or 1/2 capsule daily, every two weeks increase dose by 1/2 scoop or 1/2 capsule until 6 scoops or capsules are reached. Continue 6 scoops/capsules for 90 days (www.GardenofLife.com).
- Lactobacillus GG, also known as Culturelle, by VRP (www.lactobacillusgg.com).

Appendix V - Gluten and Casein Free Diet

- Start with **one at a time:**
    - o Try casein-free for three weeks
    - o Then remove gluten and continue both for three months
- Substitute same foods child likes with gluten/casein-free options. For example, if they eat waffles every morning, buy rice flour waffles from Trader Joe's.
- Give it time. A child may refuse to eat for a few days (because of withdrawals or as a control tactic) but if you hold out, most often he or she will come around. However, if you become concerned, consult a professional. While uncommon, it is not unheard of that an ASD child ends up in the hospital from refusing food.
- Try some prepared foods and mixes either from a natural food store or the Internet.
- For younger kids, just make the changes. Put gluten and dairy free options in the old containers, i.e. put rice milk in the milk container.
  For older children or children that know it's not the "real" thing, explain how their ailments will improve by doing this.
- For consumption of wheat and dairy try Houston Nutraceuticals Peptizyde (or AFP Peptizyde) which addresses these two food groups specifically.
- Be sure to quiz restaurants, vendors, manufacturers, etc very carefully. If you are still uncertain or can't get good information, don't eat their products.
- If possible, work with a professional such as a physician, naturopathic doctor, or nutrition consultant who understands gluten and casein-free diets.

Once the diet is followed without infraction, it typically takes a minimum of three weeks to get the casein antibodies out of the system and three to six months for gluten. Since it often takes a while to get the hang of the GFCF diet and infractions are to be expected, I typically recommend six months on the GFCF diet before judging its effectiveness. I have seen many clients who stated that they "tried" the GFCF diet and it was not helpful, and after we have worked together on a strict GFCF diet, they saw improvement. Often the biggest problems parents have that prevent them from seeing results on GFCF are trace ingredients, incomplete understanding of gluten- and casein-containing foods, and caregiver infractions. Most people (understandably) are unaware that trace ingredients do not have to be listed on the label, such as the dusting of potatoes with a gluten flour in processing. Soy cheese often contains caseinate (casein), and malt sweetener contains gluten. Also, additional caregivers such as a grandparent, teacher, or babysitter may offer a gluten- or casein-containing food to the child.

Gluten and Dairy: Foods to Avoid and Better Choices

AVOID		BETTER CHOICES
GLUTEN	• Wheat • Oats • Rye • Spelt • Kamut • Barley • Bulgar • Baked goods • Biscuits • Bread crumbs • Breads • Breakfast cereals	• Candy • Crackers • Dumplings • Macaroni/Pasta • Malt and malt sweetener • Salad dressing • Sauces • Soups (cream) • Stuffing • Bologna and hot dogs	• Amaranth • Millet • Quinoa • Brown Rice (or white) • Kasha (Buckwheat) • Corn • Non-gluten flour for baking (buckwheat, garbanzo, rice flour) • Non-wheat pasta (corn, rice, soba noddles (buckwheat)) • Non-gluten bread (millet, rice bread) • Mochi (chewy rice baked item)
DAIRY	• Cow's milk and all cow milk products • All cheese • Yogurt • Ice cream • Cottage cheese • Cream cheese • Goat's milk and all goat milk products • Sour Cream • Butter • Whipped cream • Lactose-treated milk • Cream	• Casein (often in soy cheeses) • Caseinate • Whey • Lactose • Buttermilk • Cocoa • Condensed, powdered or evaporated milk • "Nondairy" substitutes such as Coffee-Mate • Cool Whip • Acidophilus milk	• Rice milk • Almond or hazelnut milk • Homemade nut milk • Coconut milk • Potato milk • Homemade ice cream with nut milk or coconut milk • Rice milk ice cream • Pudding made with rice or nut milk

FOOD/INGREDIENTS THAT CONTAIN GLUTEN - AVOID

- Abyssinian Hard (Wheat triticum durum)
- Alcohol (Spirits)
- Barley Grass (can contain seeds)
- Barley Hordeum vulgare
- Barley Malt
- Beer
- Bleached Flour
- Blue Cheese (made with bread)
- Bran
- Bread Flour
- Brewer's Yeast
- Brown Flour
- Bulgur (Bulgar Wheat/Nuts)
- Bulgur Wheat
- Calcium Caseinate (Contains MSG)
- Cereal Binding
- Chilton
- Club Wheat (Triticum aestivum subspecies compactum)
- Coloring
- Common Wheat (Triticum aestivum)
- Couscous
- Dextrimaltose
- Durum wheat (Triticum durum)
- Edible Starch
- Einkorn (Triticum monococcum)
- Emmer (Triticum dicoccon)
- Farina Graham
- Filler
- Food Starch
- Fu (dried wheat gluten)
- Germ
- Glutamate (Free)*
- Glutamic Acid*
- Graham Flour
- Granary Flour
- Gravy Cubes
- Groats (barley, wheat)
- Ground Spices*
- Gum Base
- Hard Wheat
- Inulin
- Kamut (Pasta wheat)
- Malt
- Malt Extract
- Malt Syrup
- Malt Flavoring
- Malt Vinegar
- Miso*
- Macha Wheat (Triticum aestivum)
- Matzo Semolina
- Mustard Powder*
- Oriental Wheat (Triticum turanicum)
- Pasta
- Pearl Barley
- Persian Wheat (Triticum carthlicum)
- Poulard Wheat (Triticum turgidum)
- Polish Wheat (Triticum polonicum)
- Rice Malt (contains barley or Koji)
- Rye
- Seitan
- Semolina
- Semolina Triticum
- Shot Wheat (Triticum aestivum)
- Soba Noodles
- Sodium Caseinate (Contains MSG)
- Soy Sauce
- Spirits (Specific Types)
- Spelt (Triticum spelta)
- Sprouted Wheat or Barley
- Stock Cubes*
- Strong Flour
- Suet in Packets
- Tabbouleh
- Teriyaki Sauce
- Textured Vegetable Protein - TVP
- Timopheevi Wheat (Triticum timopheevii)
- Triticale X triticosecale
- Udon (wheat noodles)
- Vavilovi Wheat (Triticum aestivum)
- Vegetable Starch
- Vitamins*
- Wheat Triticum aestivum
- Wheat Nuts
- Wheat, Abyssinian Hard triticum durum
- Wheat, Bulgur
- Wheat Durum Triticum
- Wheat Triticum Monococcum
- Wheat Germ (oil)
- Wheat Grass (can contain seeds)
- Whole-Meal Flour
- Wild Einkorn (Triticum boeotictim)
- Wild Emmer (Triticum dicoccoides)

FOOD/INGREDIENTS THAT _May or May not_ CONTAIN GLUTEN		
• Artificial Color*	• Hydrolyzed Plant Protein*	• Mono and Diglycerides*
• Artificial Flavoring*	• Hydrolyzed Vegetable	• Monosodium Glutimate
• Caramel Color*	Protein*	(MSG)*
• Citric Acid*	• Maltodextrin*	• Natural Flavoring*
• Dextrins*	• Modified Food Starch*	• Starch*
• Flavoring*	• Modified Starch*	• Wheat Starch

* May be problematic for other reasons

Source: GFCFDiet.com - Read Special Diets for Special Kids, I and II.

Appendix VI – Parents Ratings of Interventions

ARI Publ. 34/March 2009

PARENT RATINGS OF BEHAVIORAL EFFECTS OF BIOMEDICAL INTERVENTIONS
Autism Research Institute • 4182 Adams Avenue • San Diego, CA 92116

The parents of autistic children represent a vast and important reservoir of information on the benefits—and adverse effects—of the large variety of drugs and other interventions that have been tried with their children. Since 1967 the Autism Research Institute has been collecting parent ratings of the usefulness of the many interventions tried on their autistic children.

The following data have been collected from the more than 27,000 parents who have completed our questionnaires designed to collect such information. For the purposes of the present table, the parents responses on a six-point scale have been combined into three categories: "made worse" (ratings 1 and 2), "no effect" (ratings 3 and 4), and "made better" (ratings 5 and 6). The "Better:Worse" column gives the number of children who "Got Better" for each one who "Got Worse."

DRUGS	Got Worse[A]	No Effect	Got Better	Better:Worse	No. of Cases[B]
Actos	19%	60%	21%	1.1:1	140
Aderall	43%	26%	31%	0.7:1	894
Amphetamine	47%	28%	25%	0.5:1	1355
Anafranil	32%	39%	29%	1.1:1	440
Antibiotics	33%	50%	18%	0.5:1	2507
Antifungals[C]					
Diflucan	5%	34%	62%	13:1	1214
Nystatin	5%	43%	52%	11:1	1969
Atarax	26%	53%	21%	0.8:1	543
Benadryl	24%	50%	26%	1.1:1	3230
Beta Blocker	18%	51%	31%	1.7:1	306
Buspar	29%	42%	28%	1.0:1	431
Chloral Hydrate	42%	39%	19%	0.5:1	498
Clonidine	22%	32%	46%	2.1:1	1658
Clozapine	38%	43%	19%	0.5:1	170
Cogentin	20%	53%	27%	1.4:1	198
Cylert	45%	35%	19%	0.4:1	634
Depakene[D]					
Behavior	25%	44%	31%	1.2:1	1146
Seizures	12%	33%	55%	4.6:1	761
Desipramine	34%	35%	32%	0.9:1	95
Dilantin[D]					
Behavior	28%	49%	23%	0.8:1	1127
Seizures	16%	37%	47%	3.0:1	454
Fenfluramine	21%	52%	27%	1.3:1	483
Haldol	38%	28%	34%	0.9:1	1222
IVIG	7%	39%	54%	7.6:1	142
Klonapin[D]					
Behavior	31%	40%	29%	0.9:1	270
Seizures	29%	55%	16%	0.6:1	86
Lithium	22%	48%	31%	1.4:1	515
Luvox	31%	37%	32%	1.0:1	251
Mellaril	29%	38%	33%	1.2:1	2108
Mysoline[D]					
Behavior	41%	46%	13%	0.3:1	156
Seizures	21%	55%	24%	1.1:1	85
Naltrexone Low Dose Naltrexone	11%	52%	38%	4.0:1	190
Paxil	34%	32%	35%	1.0:1	471
Phenobarb.[D]					
Behavior	48%	37%	16%	0.3:1	1125
Seizures	18%	44%	38%	2.2:1	543
Prolixin	30%	41%	28%	0.9:1	109
Prozac	33%	32%	35%	1.1:1	1391
Risperidal	21%	26%	54%	2.6:1	1216
Ritalin	45%	26%	29%	0.6:1	4256
Secretin					
Intravenous	7%	50%	43%	6.4:1	597
Transderm.	9%	56%	35%	3.9:1	257
Stelazine	29%	45%	26%	0.9:1	437
Steroids	34%	30%	36%	1.1:1	204
Tegretol[D]					
Behavior	25%	45%	30%	1.2:1	1556
Seizures	14%	33%	53%	3.8:1	872
Thorazine	36%	40%	24%	0.7:1	945
Tofranil	30%	38%	32%	1.1:1	785
Valium	35%	42%	24%	0.7:1	895
Valtrex	8%	42%	50%	6.7:1	238
Zarontin[D]					
Behavior	34%	48%	18%	0.5:1	164
Seizures	20%	55%	25%	1.2:1	125
Zoloft	35%	33%	31%	0.9:1	579

BIOMEDICAL/ NON-DRUG/ SUPPLEMENTS	Got Worse[A]	No Effect	Got Better	Better:Worse	No. of Cases[B]
Calcium[E]	3%	60%	36%	11:1	2832
Cod Liver Oil	4%	41%	55%	14:1	2550
Cod Liver Oil with Bethanecol	11%	53%	36%	3.4:1	203
Colostrum	6%	56%	38%	6.8:1	851
Detox. (Chelation)[C]	3%	23%	74%	24:1	1382
Digestive Enzymes	3%	35%	62%	19:1	2350
DMG	8%	50%	42%	5.3:1	6363
Fatty Acids	2%	39%	59%	31:1	1680
5 HTP	11%	42%	47%	4.2:1	644
Folic Acid	5%	50%	45%	10:1	2505
Food Allergy Trtmnt	2%	31%	67%	27:1	1294
Hyperbaric Oxygen Therapy	5%	30%	65%	12:1	219
Magnesium	6%	65%	29%	4.6:1	301
Melatonin	8%	26%	66%	8.3:1	1687
Methyl B12 (nasal)	10%	45%	44%	4.2:1	240
Methyl B12 (subcut.)	6%	22%	72%	12:1	899
MT Promoter	8%	47%	44%	5.5:1	99
P5P (Vit. B6)	11%	40%	48%	4.3:1	920
Pepcid	11%	57%	32%	2.9:1	220
SAMe	16%	62%	23%	1.4:1	244
St. Johns Wort	19%	64%	18%	0.9:1	217
TMG	16%	43%	41%	2.6:1	1132
Transfer Factor	8%	47%	45%	5.9:1	274
Vitamin A	3%	54%	44%	16:1	1535
Vitamin B3	4%	51%	45%	10:1	1192
Vit. B6/Mag.	4%	46%	49%	11:1	7256
Vitamin C	2%	52%	46%	20:1	3077
Zinc	2%	44%	54%	24:1	2738
SPECIAL DIETS					
Candida Diet	3%	39%	58%	21:1	1141
Feingold Diet	2%	40%	58%	26:1	1041
Gluten-/Casein- Free Diet	3%	28%	69%	24:1	3593
Low Oxalate Diet	7%	43%	50%	6.8:1	164
Removed Chocolate	2%	46%	52%	28:1	2264
Removed Eggs	2%	53%	45%	20:1	1658
Removed Milk Products/Dairy	2%	44%	55%	32:1	6950
Removed Sugar	2%	46%	52%	27:1	4589
Removed Wheat	2%	43%	55%	30:1	4340
Rotation Diet	2%	43%	55%	23:1	1097
Specific Carbo- hydrate Diet	7%	22%	71%	10:1	537

A. "Worse" refers only to worse behavior. Drugs, but not nutrients, typically also cause physical problems if used long-term.
B. No. of cases is cumulative over several decades, so does not reflect current usage levels (e.g., Haldol is now seldom used).
C. Antifungal drugs and chelation are used selectively, where evidence indicates they are needed.
D. Seizure drugs: top line behavior effects, bottom line effects on seizures
E. Calcium effects are not due to dairy-free diet; statistics are similar for milk drinkers and non-milk drinkers.

Appendix VII - Phenol Protocol

The following is the protocol I created for phenols--it is an approach that includes:

1) A low phenol diet. I often use the Feingold Diet to start. Other choices include the Failsafe Diet, Sarah's Diet or some version of removing salicylates, phenols, amines, glutamates, etc. While these other diets are removing more than just phenol, they are often further restrictions that are sometimes necessary.

2) Supplements and substances that add sulfate to aid sulfation

3) Enzymes to help break down remaining phenols.

As phenols cannot ever be completely eliminated, the key is determining the amount of phenols that are tolerated (at a given time, or in a day) for an individual. Think of phenol processing like water going through a funnel: at a certain amount, the body can no longer process them and you will be overloaded (overflowing). This can change based on what else is happening at a given time, for example, if the funnel is becoming clogged with other substances (the body is clogged with other toxins or requires sulfate for other processing) the body may be more sensitive or overloaded on a particular day.

Determination of Phenol Sensitivity

Currently, there is no one test to directly determine phenol sensitivity or faulty sulfation. I use a combination of physical, biochemical, behavioral, and cognitive signs/symptoms:

- Reactions to phenol/salicylates
- Unusual cravings for phenolic foods
- Family history of related neurological and other medical disorders
- A phase two liver detox test for sulfation
- Levels of sulfate in the blood versus urine
- Levels of metabolites of methionine cascade.

What Interferes with Sulfation

- Low sulfate levels
- Chlorine (pools and water supply)
- Mercury or other heavy metals

Symptoms of Phenol Sensitivity

- Dark circles under eyes
- Red face/ears
- Diarrhea
- Hyperactivity
- Impulsivity
- Aggression
- Headache
- Head banging/self-injury, impatience
- Short attention span
- Difficulty falling asleep
- Night waking for several hours.
- Inappropriate laughter
- Hives or rashes
- Itchy skin
- Asthma and breathing difficulties
- Mouth ulcers
- Excessive thirst (normal urination)
- Odorous bed clothes
- Dyslexia
- Speech difficulties
- Tics
- Some forms of seizures
- Bedwetting and day wetting
- Swelling of hands and feet
- Persistent cough
- Stomachache

Common Familial Disorders

I often consider the family history of the child when suspecting a phenol intolerance. If it there a lot of neurological and/or autoimmune conditions in a family, I begin to explore further if evidence support a possible sulfation insufficiency. If sulfation is poor, the ability to process phenols is greatly reduced and reactions are likely.

Improving Processing of Phenols

Process or breakdown phenols by using:
- Houston Nutraceuticals – No-Fenol breaks down phenols, and sometimes HN-Zyme Prime can help. (www.houstonni.com).
- Molybdenum can help process phenols.

Supplement with sulfate (building blocks):
- <u>Topically absorb through skin:</u>
  - **Epsom Salt** Bath (which is magnesium salt) (1/2-2 cups per bath, very warm – as warm as is comfortable). Soak 20 minutes. May only be able to start with 1 T if sensitive or if hyperactivity results. You can leave salt residue on body if not itchy or irritating. Some (including Pangborn and Baker) recommend adding ¼ of baking soda to the bath.
  - **Epsom Salt Foot Soaks** (Epsom salt) work for some children.
  - **Lotion** (from Karen D. on www.enzymestuff.com)
    Heat 1 teaspoon of water and add 3 tablespoons of Epsom salts. To this, add 4 ounces of any lotion that is fragrance free and as natural as possible. Often a thicker lotion will make the lotion easier to use.
  - **Cream** (recipe by Mary Kaye, not Mary Kay Cosmetics).
    - o   1 cup epsom salt
    - o   2 tsp non-aluminum baking soda
    - o   1/2 cup boiling distilled water
    - o   2 T glycerin
    - o   1/4 almond, olive or sunflower oil
    - o   1/2 cup favorite natural lotion or cream or 1/2 cup coconut butter
    - o   a few drops lavender essential oil (organic) or other essential oil (optional)
    - o   1 T flaxseed oil
    - o   1 T evening primrose oil
    - o   1 T MSM powder (to boost sulfates)

    Blend at high speed adding ingredients a little at a time. Boil water and add to Epsom salt and baking soda in blender, pulse until dissolved and not grainy (must be boiling). Add glycerin, then slowly add oils while blending to emulsify. Still blending add lotion, cream or coconut butter a little at a time. Pour into a clean container, preferably ceramic or glass. If it separates into layers when cool, rewarm and add 2 tablespoons of guar gum dissolved into a bit of hot water, reblend and cool.

Sulfate taken orally:

- MSM
- NAC
- Glucosamine sulfate
- N-Acetyl Glucosamine
- Multivitamin that contains sulfate: Brainchild Nutritionals
- Intestimend: Emergency phenol overload
  - According to Lang, 1 oz every 3-4 hours in some juice with emergency phenol consumption. Give one dose and see if improved. May need to do 2-3 doses over 24 hour period. Use only after candida overgrowth is under control

Boost methylation

After you remove any offending phenolic substances, you can begin to boost phenol processing. This can be done by boosting methylation or sulfation with nutrients such as B12, folic acid, DMG or TMG, and B6.

Appendix VIII - Raw dairy

Dairy causes a great deal of controversy among nutrition consultants. Some say dairy products are vitally important, others say use only non-fat and low fat products, while others say the decrease in lactase enzyme in adults is evidence that we are not supposed to consume milk products past early childhood. Vegans say that cow milk is for cow, and absolutely not for humans.

With autistic spectrum disorders we know that many children react to the casein in milk. As such, most children using biomedical approaches avoid dairy. I have a couple possible reasons *why* these children have inflammation and immune responses from casein.

What people rarely consider is whether the pasteurization of milk is creating any of the current intolerances to milk, in the general population or with the autistic child. Until now, few have suggested that milk should be consumed raw, as nature intended. Why have we consumed dairy for so many generations and now it is one of the top sensitivities in the country and autistic population?

I suspect two possible reasons why raw milk is not problematic, but pasteurized is (which seems to be the experience among many families with ASD). Pasteurization heats the milk to high temperatures that may alter the molecular structure of the protein molecules, causing the body not to recognize it. This inability for the body to identify the protein could create casein intolerance and IgG response. Secondly, cows are not supposed to eat a diet high in grains—they eat grass. Unfortunately modern dairy production uses grain-fed cows. As this is not the cows' natural diet and because grains are high in lectins, it's possible that this commercial (pasteurized) milk may have an increase in inflammatory lectins from the grain in their milk, possibly contributing to gut inflammation in people who consume it.

Because the CDC and FDA and most health and government officials claim that raw milk is "dangerous" or "harmful," many states and countries do not allow for the legal sale of raw milk. I'm from California where we are lucky because raw milk and dairy products are sold in stores. I have many clients using raw milk with success. More research needs to be done but I have heard from many people—with autism and without—who cannot handle pasteurized dairy of any kind but can consume raw dairy.

Pasteurized milk is much less wholesome, as pasteurization:

- Kills the natural enzymes for easy digestion of the milk.
- Destroys virtually all the phosphatase, an enzyme that aids in the absorption of calcium (Allen, 2004).
- Kills good bacteria (that fights bad bacteria) that good for our gut.
- Reduces vitamin content and destroys vitamins A (Krauss, 1933), C, B12 and B6, essential nutrients for immune function, healing and many other systems.
- Promotes pathogens and is associated with allergies.

Pasteurized milk is not good for anyone. Calves fed pasteurized milk don't thrive and often die before adulthood. Ultra-pasteurization is even worse than standard pasteurization methods. Used to get rid of heat-resistant bacteria and give it a longer shelf life, this process takes milk from a chilled temperature to above the boiling point in less than two seconds.

On the other hand, raw milk:
- Contains many enzymes for easier digestion.
- Is rich in good bacteria.
- Is from pastured cows with milk rich in omega-3 fatty acids
- Is high in enzymes to increase digestibility as well as phosphatase for the absorption of calcium in the milk.
- Is higher in vitamins A and D, important in immune function, calcium absorption, protein assimilation, strong bones and more. It is important to note that these are the natural forms of these vitamins, not ones added in later.
- Is high in butyric acid, which nourishes the brain and intestinal lining and has antimicrobial properties.

Not all children on the autistic spectrum can handle raw milk and dairy products. In fact, many cannot, until the gut is healed, and some not at all. A good place to start is with raw butter. It contains very little casein and can sometimes be tolerated when all other dairy cannot. Also the butyric acid in the raw butter is healing.

Safety

Firstly, I would never consume *commercial* milk raw. Commercial milk comes from unhealthy cows given tons of antibiotics. These cows harbor disease resistant strains of pathogenic bacteria. However, farmers who produce raw milk take the utmost in care of their animals because this type of food and way of life is important to them.

Public health officials warn that raw milk poses the risk of transmitting bacteria such as listeria, E. coli and salmonella. Pasteurization was instituted in the 1920s to combat tuberculosis, infant diarrhea, fever and other diseases caused by poor animal nutrition and dirty production methods of mass produced milk. Pasteurization kills these bacteria while extending the milk's shelf life so that the dairy industry profits while consumers and cows suffer. With modern organically raised cows, stainless steel tanks and milking machines, refrigerated trucks and inspection methods many of the reasons for pasteurization are eliminated.

The biggest public campaign against raw milk has been based on promoting fear about raw milk's safety, so let's examine this issue more closely. The Weston A. Price Foundation Website (http://westonaprice.org) states:

"Except for a brief hiatus in 1990, raw milk has always been for sale commercially in California, usually in health food stores, although I can remember a period when it was even sold in grocery stores. Millions of people consumed commercial raw milk during that period and although the health department kept an eagle eye open for any possible evidence of harm, not a single incidence was reported. During the same period, there were many instances of contamination in pasteurized milk, some of which resulted in death."

On May 19, 2004, Mark McAfee, founder of Organic Pastures Dairy, stated:

"For the last four years, Organic Pastures Dairy has produced a full line of raw organic dairy products for retail sale (300 stores including Whole Foods) and consumption here in California. The state of California (CDFA) monitors and tests all of our raw dairy products multiple times per month. The state has never found one pathogen (salmonella, E. coli O157:H7 or listeria) in any of our products. Even more interesting is the fact that not one human pathogen has ever been found in the hundreds of environmental swabs that have been taken in our plant facility [yet] the typical conventional milk tank had either salmonella or E. coli O157:H7 detected about 30 percent of the time. In comparison, Organic Pastures has never had one pathogen – ever."

While it is certainly possible to become sick from drinking contaminated raw milk, it is also possible to become sick from almost any food source such as listeria in lunchmeat. Also, it appears that raw milk may be safer than commercial since healthy cows don't harbor bad bacteria.

I know a lot of people, including myself, who consume raw milk, raw homemade yogurt, raw butter, and raw cheese. These products taste incredible and help promote improved health.

Commercial vs. Raw vs. Organic

Much of vegans' concern over milk on is how poorly cows are treated. There is nothing natural about how commercial milk cows are raised. They are selectively bred to generate the most milk, fed a diet high in protein, kept in confined spaces, and fed antibiotics to combat poor living conditions, treatment, and disease. These cows are not naturally raised healthy animals. They pump out three to four times the amount of milk of their counterparts and die prematurely.

Cows raised for raw milk production are often old-fashioned Jersey and Guernsey cows and well taken care of. They need to be because there are no antibiotics poured into their "feed." In fact, in many cases there is no "feed" other than the pesticide-free green grass they graze one. They live outdoors to graze and therefore get plenty of sunlight. This creates an abundant amount of vitamins A & D present in the butterfat.

Be aware even cows raised for organic but pasteurized milk are often not raised on their natural diet of green grass. While organic is certainly superior to commercial milk, it is lacking many of the properties of raw milk due to pasteurization (and often homogenization).

Whole Fat Milk

The low-fat and non-fat milk recommendations made by many nutritionists of the past did not take into consideration the importance of the essential milk fatty acids and fat soluble vitamins. Even today, the vast majority of people think they are doing a good thing by consuming low fat milk. When we are talking about pasteurized milk products deficient in all of the important qualities of pasture-raised, raw dairy (the good essential fatty acids, vitamins A and D, enzymes, probiotics, and more) this may be true; however, the fat found in the milk of pastured-raised, organic raw dairy provides many essential health benefits. When consuming "real milk" you want to consume the fat it provides.

Vitamins A and D, found naturally in the fat of real milk, are needed for proper assimilation of calcium and protein. The fat in milk is rich in fatty acids, which protect against disease and stimulate the immune system. It contains glyco-spingolipids that prevent intestinal distress. It also contains conjugated linoleic acid that has strong anticancer properties and aids fat burning.

Additionally, low fat milk has powdered skim milk added, and in the process of powdering it, the cholesterol is dangerously oxidized creating a substance that is damaging to the arteries. It is not the fat in milk, but the oxidation of the cholesterol added to milk that creates heart disease. This high heat drying process also creates cross-linked proteins and nitrate compounds, which are carcinogenic. Additionally, free glutamic acid is created which is toxic to the nervous system and a big problem for many with autism, and very likely one of the many reasons milk is not tolerated by children with autistic spectrum disorders.

Digestibility

Natural enzymes, probiotics, and unadulterated proteins make raw milk much easier to digest and assimilate than commercial milk products. The process of heating the milk during pasteurization alters the protein and is believed to be one of the factors creating the high rates of casein sensitivity. While studies have not been done on this, it seems logical that the body recognizes what it has been familiar with for generations. Newly created foods may not be recognized by the immune system—and a sensitivity could result.

Milk and cheeses from raw milk contain a full array of enzymes and therefore are more easily digested. When cheese is eaten unheated it is even more digestible. In addition, when milk is fermented, casein is predigested, making digestion of casein easier.

While it is true that some populations do not continue to produce lactase (the enzyme to break down lactose and prevent lactose-intolerance) additional decline in lactase in adults is due to overuse of antibiotics and the deficiency in good bacteria that results. Raw milk and lactobacillus in fermented milk have adequate amounts of enzymes present to break down the milk for easy digestion, while pasteurization kills these enzymes and probiotics.

Raw Dairy Resources

Because of this fear that has been created again unpasteurized dairy, most states don't even sell raw dairy. If your state does not sell raw milk commercially, you can often get it from the farm, a co-op, cow share, or other non-commercial means. You can often purchase it as "pet food" in your state or have it shipped from another state at pet food. However, in some states, it is actually illegal. Check with the Weston A. Price Foundation (WestonAPrice.org) for potential resources near you.

Research

As this is such an important decision—especially for pregnant women, children, and the immune compromised—it is essential for you to do your own research to feel personally comfortable before proceeding. As it is possible to get sick from any food, which of course includes raw milk, you want to find a good source and feel comfortable before proceeding.

Unfortunately, the FDA does not allow current research on raw milk. However, there are many studies from the 1920s and 30s that provide valuable information (RealMilk.com highlights many). There was a recent study in Europe on "farm milk" that showed lower incidences of allergies and asthma with those children who consumed farm milk. (Waser, 2006) When we approached the author of the study about the type of milk, he said farm families and those in rural areas typically consume their milk raw, although the study did not confirm the use of raw dairy in all cases.

It may take many years to get more information and research on raw milk. I heard there may be a prominent Stanford researcher interested in conducting a study on raw milk. Until then, I encourage families that are having positive results from raw dairy to comment on my blog (NourishingHope.com) so we can gather anecdotal evidence to help other families.

Appendix IX - Specific Carbohydrate Diet (SCD) Summary

Foods to avoid on SCD

- No corn
- No potatoes (white or sweet)
- No grains
- No products made from grains or starches (rice or potato milk)
- No beans unless specified as allowable
- No soy products
- No molasses
- No corn syrup
- No maple syrup
- No artificial sweeteners (including sucralose or Splenda)
- No garlic and onion powder
- No pasta
- No cornstarch, arrowroot powder, tapioca, agar-agar or carrageenan
- No pectin in making jellies and jams
- No chocolate or carob
- No ketchup
- No baking powder (baking soda is fine)
- Many supplements are not allowed because of SCD non-compliant fillers

Allowable SCD foods (if no prior sensitivity)

- Meat
- Eggs
- Natural cheeses (if not casein intolerant)
- Homemade yogurt (if not casein intolerant)
- Non-starchy vegetables
- Some beans: Dried white (navy) beans, lentils, split peas, lima beans
- Fruit and 100% fruit juice not from concentrate
- Nuts
- Honey
- Nut milk
- Oils made from grains (such as corn oil and soybean oil) are permitted.
- Spices (of any kind except mixtures like apple pie spice and curry powder)
- Ghee

Appendix X - Elimination Diet

- Give up all possible food sensitivities for 10 days. These include:
  - Wheat
  - All gluten grains (oats, barley, rye, spelt, kamut) – Glutenfreeoats.com has GF oats
  - Dairy
  - Eggs
  - Soy (tofu, soy sauce, miso, tempeh)
  - Sugar (honey, maple syrup, sugar, fructose, etc.)
  - Chocolate
  - Corn
  - Citrus
  - Peanuts
  - Processed foods (containing hidden wheat and dairy)
  - Artificial ingredients (as they can mask improvement and problems)
- Add back one at a time, having a serving for breakfast and lunch.
- Wait a total of three days and record any symptoms that occur during this time. For example, headache, gas/bloating, diarrhea, constipation, poor mood, etc.
- If a reaction occurs, do not add that food back to diet and proceed to next food item.
- If you are unsure of a reaction, do not add food back yet and retest at another time.
- If no reaction is noticed and you feel great, add food back to diet and proceed to next item until all are tested.

Foods to eat During This Time

- Grains: brown rice, quinoa, amaranth, millet. Pasta, crackers and cereals made from rice.
- Breads: Gluten-free breads (found in refrigerated section of health food store), mochi (chewy baked item, made from brown rice). Rice crackers.
- Beans (any except soy): Black, pinto, refried beans, garbanzo, hummus, lentils.
- Vegetables: all except corn.
- Root vegetables and squash: potatoes (but avoid potato chips and fries unless confirmed gluten-free), sweet potatoes, yams, butternut squash.
- Fruit, except citrus.
- Meat: Turkey, chicken, beef, pork, buffalo.
- Fish: any.
- Nuts and seeds and nut butters: any except soy and peanuts.

Appendix XI – Salicylates in Foods

Salicylates in foods/100 g
Swain et al*

Negligible	Low 0.1-0.25 mg	Moderate 0.25—0.49 mg	High 0.5—1.0 mg	Very high > 1.0 mg
Vegetables				
Bamboo shoots Brussels sprouts Cabbage Celery Chive Dried beans Dried peas Green beans Green peas Leek Lentils Lettuce (Iceberg) Mungbean sprouts Potato, peeled white Red cabbage Shallots Swedes	Asparagus, fresh Beetroot Carrot, fresh Cauliflower Choko Corn on the cob Mushroom, fresh Onion Potato, white, un- peeled Pumpkin Tomato, fresh Turnip	Asparagus, canned Beetroot, canned Corn niblets, canned Chinese vegetables Lettuce (other) Marrow Olives, black, can Parsley Parsnip Potato (new, red) Pumpkin Snow peas Snow pea sprouts Sweet corn Sweet potato, yellow	Alfalfa Artichoke Broad beans Broccoli Chili, green, yellow Corn, creamed Cucumber Eggplant Fava beans Okra Spinach, fresh Squash Sweet potato, white Tomato, canned Water chestnut Watercress	Broad bean Capsicum, green Champignon, canned Chilli, red Chicory Endive Gherkin Green Pepper Mushroom, canned Olives, green, canned Radish Tomato, any concen- trate, sauce Zucchini
Fruit				
Banana Pear, peeled	Apple, golden & red delicious Fig, kadota Cherries, sour can Grapes, green, can Lemon, fresh Mango Pawpaw Passionfruit Plum, green, fresh Persimmon Pineapple juice Rhubarb Tamarillo	Apple, Jonathan, fresh Apple, canned Ard- mona® Grapefruit juice Kiwi Lychee Loquat Nectarine, fresh Pear, with peel Plum Watermelon	Apple, Granny Smith Avocado, fresh Cherries Fig, calamata, dried Grapes, red Grape juice Grapefruit, fresh Mandarin, fresh Mulberry Peach, fresh, canned Tangelo, fresh	Apricots Blackberries Blueberries Boysenberries Cantaloupe Cherries, canned Cranberry sauce and canned Currants Dates Grapes, fresh Guava Loganberries Orange Pineapple Prunes, Raisins Raspberries Strawberries Sultanas Youngberry

* Swain AR, et al., "Salicylates in Foods." *J Am Diet Assoc*. 1985 Aug;85(8):950-60.

Nuts and Seeds				
Cashews	Pecans Peanut butter Poppy seeds Sesame seeds Hazelnuts Sunflower seeds	Coconut, desiccated Brazil nuts	Pine nuts Macadamia nuts Pistachio nuts	Almonds Peanuts Water chestnuts
Seasonings				
Garlic Parsley Chives Coriander, fresh leaves	Vinegar Soy sauce Saffron Tandori spice powder Horseradish, can	Fennel	Vegemite	All other Extremely high: Allspice Aniseed **Canella** Cayenne Celery Cinnamon **Cumin** **Curry powder** **Dill, dry** Fenugreek Five spice **Garam masala** Ginger Mace Mint Mixed herbs Mustard **Oregano** **Paprika, hot** Paprika, sweet Pepper **Rosemary** Sage Tarragon **Turmeric** **Thyme** Worcestershire sauce
Sweets and sugars				
Pascalls cream caramel® Golden syrup Maple syrup White sugar	Molasses Brown sugar		Honey	Licorice Peppermints **Honey**
Beverages				
Cocoa powder Carob powder Ovaltine® Ecco cereal coffee®	Chamomile tea	Coffee, Instant Rosehip tea (herbal) Fruit tea (herbal)		**Tea**, all varieties
Alcoholic beverages				
	Vodka, Whiskey, Gin	Brandy, Vermouth	Sherry Cointreau® Tia Maria®	Liqueur Rum Champagne, Wines

* from http://users.bigpond.net.au/allergydietitian/fi/img37.gif

195

Appendix XII - Feingold Diet

Foods Eliminated of Phase I of Feingold Diet

Salicylates	Phenols and other additives
• Almonds	• BHA, BHT – synthetic antioxidant
• Apples	• Preservatives
• Apricots	• Anticaking agents
• Aspirin	• Artificial colors
• Berries, raspberries, cherries	• Artificial flavoring
• Chili powder	• Artificial preservatives
• Cider and cider vinegar	• Benzoates
• Cloves	• Corn syrup
• Coffee	• Emulsifiers
• Cola drinks	• Hydrolyzed vegetable protein
• Cucumbers and pickles	• Mineral salts
• Curry powder	• MSG
• Endive	• Nitrates
• Grapes, raisins, currants	• Nitrites
• Honey	• Perfumes
• Nectarines and peaches	• Sorbates
• Oil of wintergreen	• Sulfites
• Oranges and oranges	
• Paprika	
• Peppers (bell and chili)	
• Pineapple	
• Plums and prunes	
• Radishes	
• Tea	
• Tomatoes	
• Wine and wine vinegar	

ACCEPTABLE FOODS FOR FEINGOLD/MOST ARE LOW SALICYLATE	
FRUITS	**VEGETABLES**
• Pears	• Artichokes
• Lemon/lime	• Asparagus
• Grapefruit	• Alfalfa
• Mango	• Bamboo
• Papaya	• Beans
• Pineapple (not fresh)	• Beets
• Persimmon	• Broccoli
• Pomegranate	• Cabbage
• Kiwi	• Carrots
• Dates	• Cauliflower
• Figs	• Celery
• Melon	• Corn
• Honeydew melon	• Eggplant
• Watermelon	• Green/String beans
• Cantaloupe	• Leafy greens
• Avocado	• Lettuce
• Guava	• Lentils
• Coconut	• Mushrooms
• Kumquat	• Okra
• Loquat	• Olives
• Starfruit	• Parsley
	• Parsnips
	• Peas
	• Potatoes
	• Radishes
	• Rhubarb
	• Rutabaga
	• Sorrel
	• Spinach
	• Squash
	• Sweet potatoes
	• Turnips
	• Water chestnuts
	• Watercress

Appendix XIII - Failsafe Diet

Failsafe Diet includes the removal of the full range of salicylates (not just the Feingold ones); amines such as: histamine, phenylethylamine, serotonin, tyramine, dopamine; and free glutamate. Amines occur naturally in food, and are released in higher quantities when broken down by fermentation. As you can see, there are many fermented foods that are high amines. Additionally, cooking and aging meats leads to higher levels of amines, so meat should be as fresh as possible, and not slow-cooked, aged, or fermented.

Whether someone should eat these foods (as raw sauerkraut and others can be healing for the gut) or avoid them (because of amine sensitivity), can be confusing and difficult to determine. There is a test, the LEAP test (NOWLEAP.com) that can test for tyramine and phenylethylamine sensitivity. This may be a helpful way to determine whether to consume or avoid those foods.

Amines to Avoid		
Tyramine	**Phenylethylamine**	**Histamine**
<ul><li>Cheese, aged</li><li>Fruit, overripe and dehydrated</li><li>Meats, aged and processed</li><li>Red wine or beer</li><li>Sauerkraut</li><li>Smoked, cured or pickled meat or fish</li><li>Soy sauce, miso, tempeh</li><li>Yeast extracts</li></ul>	<ul><li>Cheese, aged</li><li>Chocolate</li><li>Citric acid</li><li>Citrus fruit</li><li>Cocoa</li><li>Red wine</li></ul>	<ul><li>Avocado</li><li>Beer</li><li>Cheese, especially aged</li><li>Chicken liver</li><li>Chocolate</li><li>Citrus fruit</li><li>Eggplant</li><li>Pineapple</li><li>Pork</li><li>Processed meat, such as salami, sausage, hotdog</li><li>Sauerkraut</li><li>Smoked and canned fish</li><li>Spinach</li><li>Strawberry</li><li>Tofu, tempeh, miso, tamari</li><li>Tomato, tomato sauce, tomato paste</li><li>Vinegar and vinegar containing condiments</li><li>Wine, red wine, and champagne</li><li>Yeast and foods containing yeast</li></ul>

Additional amines avoided on the Failsafe diet:

Banana	Plums/prunes	Mushrooms
Bone broths	Black walnut	Broccoli
Slow-cooked meats	Coconut	Cauliflower
Aged meats	Peanut	Raspberry
Grapes/rasisins	Pecan	Pineapple

Free Glutamates to Avoid	
Food	Free glutamate (mg/100g)
Kombu seaweed	2240
Marmite	1960
Vegemite	1431
Nori seaweed	1378
Roquefort cheese	1280
Parmesan cheese	1200
Chinese soy sauce	1090
Japanese soy sauce	782
Cured ham	337
Grape juice	258
Peas	200
Tomatoes	140
Corn	130

Additional foods high in free glutamate are:

- Broccoli
- Mushrooms
- Grapes/raisins
- Plums/prune
- Processed lunch meats, salami, and sausage
- Miso and tempeh
- Hydrolyzed vegetable protein
- Gravies, stock cubes
- Yeast extracts
- Sauerkraut

Appendix XIV - Low Oxalate Diet (LOD)

The use of the low oxalate diet has been spearheaded by Susan Owens, a brilliant researcher on sulfur chemistry, autism, and the LOD. Normally, a healthy gut will not absorb too many oxalates (naturally occurring in high levels in certain foods) from the diet because they are metabolized by the good bacteria in the gut or bound to minerals and excreted in the stool.

However, when the gut is leaky these oxalates are absorbed and high levels ending up in the blood, urine, and tissues (especially damaged tissue). This absorption creates inflammation and pain and contributes to inflammation in the intestines and leaky gut. This is a situation that perpetuates leaky gut. In cells, oxalates can lead to oxidative damage, depletion of glutathione, immune system's inflammatory cycle, and pain. The calcium oxalate crystals are sharp and the pain can be debilitating. I had a friend with shoulder inflammation who developed calcium oxalate crystals in her shoulder. The pain was so great she was unable to sleep for two days until she sought some initial relief from a doctor. (Once diagnosed with "calcium crystals," she implemented the low oxalate diet and it is began to help immediately.)

Oxalates create other challenges as well. Look at this list below from Owens that really helps paint a picture that is consistent with many of the symptoms/imbalances we see with autistic spectrum disorders. Oxalates can (from http://health.groups.yahoo.com/group/Trying_Low_Oxalates/):
*   Induce oxidative stress
*   Lower glutathione levels and increasing oxidized glutathione
*   Tie up sulfur chemistry
*   Pull sulfate out of cells
*   Shift immune system to TH2
*   Cause histamine release
*   Impair growth and sugar regulation
*   Tie up calcium and iron
*   Lead to intestinal migraine
*   Impair growth

The body gets oxalate through consuming foods containing oxalate and/or by manufacturing it.

Low thiamine and pantothenic acid, and high glycine and vitamin C can cause the body to product excess oxalates. Additionally aspergillus and penicillium (and possibly candida), as well as human metabolism create oxalates. Related to sulfur chemistry, when B6 is low, oxalate levels increase and sulfur chemistry decreases. Additionally, according to Owens, when sulfur is deficient, it becomes extremely difficult to keep the body from making excess oxalates. Oxalate and sulfate share transport into the cell—when sulfate is low, oxalate can cross into cells (potentially gumming up cellular processes and mitochondrial function).

Lactobacillus acidophilus is an "oxalating-eating" microorganism, but according to Susan Owens, when oxalates are in excess lactobacillus can be killed off. Owens questions whether this is why certain children have a very difficult time colonizing and building lactobacillus acidophilus levels in the gut. I assume the flip side may also be true. That is, if they do not have the good bacteria levels to reduce oxalate levels, low or imbalanced flora status can lead to high levels of oxalates in the body and the corresponding challenges that result.

Interestingly, many clinicians recommend reducing intake of calcium rich foods when on a low oxalate diet as calcium binds to oxalates and appears in the crystals. Therefore they believe calcium adds to the problem. In fact, I had an adult client on a low oxalate for kidney stones and she was specifically told to pay special attention to avoiding high calcium foods and supplements. Unfortunately, this is old and inaccurate information. Calcium is both good and necessary because it binds to oxalates, but it is important to take it before meals to bind to oxalates to prevent absorption (timing is important). Fat digestion is important as undigested fat can tie up calcium. Additionally, calcium is important to preventing leaky gut as calcium is necessary for the "gatekeeping" system of nutrient absorption.

Organic acid tests can check for the presence of oxalic acid (oxalates) and other markers that might indicate that someone is having difficulty with oxalates. However, urinary oxalic acid testing has not been around for long enough for us to understand the accuracy of this test and the clicnial significance of these results and for reference ranges to be estabilished. For example, one doctor has found that children with really low levels of oxalic acid did very well on the low oxalate diet. Also, family history with oxalate kidney stones or other oxalate crystals is very telling for the potential of oxalate issue; although, this is not necessary and often not present.

Improvements:
Parents are beginning to gather data on how this diet has positively impacted their children. Experience and advice are available on the Trying_low_oxalates Yahoo group (http://health.groups.yahoo.com/group/Trying_Low_Oxalates/). Improvements have been seen in the areas of social/behavioral, gastrointestinal, physical, and urinary issues, including improvements in energy, motor skills, cognition, as well as in yeast overgrowth and other digestive symptoms. Most of these children were already on restrictive diets such as GFCF and SCD, and LOD often clears up additional issues not addressed on these other diets. Be aware that initially there may be a negative reaction (for the first several days to couple weeks) while the stored oxalates are being eliminated.

Supplements
- Add probiotics and probiotic-rich (fermented) foods to the diet—good bacteria have enzymes that breakdown oxalates.
- Calcium citrate binds to oxalates to be excreted in the stool (and not absorbed into the blood stream).
- Magnesium citrate is depleted by oxalates and may bind oxalates.
- Vitamins A and E, selenium, and arginine reduce oxalate damage.
- B6 is a cofactor for an enzyme that degrades oxalates.
- VSL#3 is the probiotic of choice according to Trying_Low_Oxalate Yahoo group.
- Reduce vitamin C to 150-250 mg per day as it can convert to oxalates.
- It appears that Vitamin K may help manage calcium and control endogenous oxalate production. More needs to be studied on this but many children are now taking vitamin K with this diet.

What to eat:

Focus on low oxalate foods and avoid high oxalate foods. However, be careful to reduce high oxalate foods slowly over time (weeks to months) especially when the individual has been on an extremely high oxalate diet in the past. Increase intake of omega-3 in the form of fish or cod liver oil. However, be aware that if fats are poorly absorbed due to bile salt deficiency, these fatty acids will bind to calcium and reduce calcium availability for binding oxalates. Signs of fat malabsorption include: diarrhea, malodorous flatulence (foul smelling gas), abdominal bloating, and increased amounts of fat in the stool (steatorrhea). Fatty stools typically are large in volume, malodorous (foul smelling), greasy, light tan or light grey in color, and tend to float in the toilet bowl. If fat absorption is low, taurine may help stimulate bile salt production. Choose meat from grass-fed (pastured) animals, as grain-fed animals (the primary type of meat sold in the U.S.) are fed soy and corn and the meat is higher in arachidonic acid possibly increasing oxalate problems. Choose fruits, vegetables, seeds, and grains low (or medium) in oxalates.

Below are lists of high and low oxalate foods. As quantity affects the amount of oxalate in a food, certain foods have a portion size included to keep them within the appropriate range.

HIGH OXALATE FOODS	LOW OXALATE FOODS
Almonds	Apple juice
Amaranth	Acorn squash
Beans, navy	Alfalfa sprouts
Beans, white	Aloe vera juice
Beer lager draft, Tuborg, Pilsner	Apples, peeled red
Beets, greens	Avocado
Beets, root	Bacon (up to 9 strips)
Bell pepper, green	Basil, fresh (1 tsp)
Black currants	Beef
Black raspberries	Butter
Breakfast cereal (bran high fiber)	Cabbage
Buckwheat	Cantaloupe
Carrots, raw	Casaba melon
Celery	Catsup
Chard	Cauliflower
Chia seeds	Cheese
Chicory, raw	Cherries, bing and sour
Chili peppers	Cherry juice
Chocolate milk	Chicken
Chocolate, plain	Chives
Cinnamon, ground >1 1/2 tsp	Cider
Cocoa	Coconut
Cocoa, dry powder	Corned beef, canned
Currants, red	Cornstarch (1 tbsp)
Dandelion greens	Cranberries, canned (Ocean Spray)*

Dark chocolate candy	Cucumbers, peeled
Escarole	Egg noodles
Figs, dried	Eggs
Fruit cocktail	Endive
Fruit salad (canned)	Fish, haddock, plaice, and flounder
Fruitcake (1 slice)	Grape juice (red and white)
Ginger (1 tbsp)	Grapefruit juice
Gooseberries	Grapes green
Graham crackers	Green peas, frozen
Graham flour	Ham
Grapes, Concord	Hamburger
Grits, white corn	Honey (1 tbsp)
Hazelnut	Honeydew
Hemp milk	Huckleberries
Juices containing berries high in oxalates	Kukicha twig tea
Kamut	Kumquat
Kiwi	Lamb
Leeks	Lemons and limes
Nuts	Lettuce, iceberg (1/2 cup)
Okra	Lychee
Olives, green (10 large)	Mangoes
Orange peel	Maple syrup, pure (1 tbsp)
Parsley	Melons
Parsnips	Milk
Peanut butter	Mung bean sprouts
Peanuts	Mustard
Pecans	Mustard, Dijon (1 tbsp)
Pepper (in excess of 1 tsp per day)	Nectarines
Peppers, green (whole)	Noodles
Pesticides (may be high)	Nutmeg
Pistachio	Nutmeg, dry (1 tsp)
Pokeweed	Oils
Potato chips (1 cup)	Onions
Potatoes, fried, boiled or baked	Orange juice
Potatoes, sweet	Oregano, dried (1 tsp)
Raspberries, red	Passion fruit
Refried beans	Peas fresh green
Rhubarb	Pepper, red
Rutabagas	Peppermint
Sesame seeds	Pineapple juice
Sorrel	Plums (green or yellow)
Soy and soy foods	Popcorn (1 cup)
Soybean curd (tofu)	Pork

Spelt	Poultry
Spinach	Raisins, golden
Star fruit	Red currant juice
Stone ground flour	Rice breakfast cereal
Swiss chard	Rice, white
Tahini	Rice, wild
Tamarillo	Rye bread
Tempeh	Sage
Turnip greens	Salt
Wheat bran (1 T)	Seafood
Wheat germ (1 T)	Sugar
Whole wheat flour (1/2 cup)	Thompson seedless, green
Yams	Turkey
Yellow Dock	Turnips, roots
Yucca root	Vanilla
	Vanilla extract
	Vinegar
	Vinegar, apple cider
	Water chestnuts
	Watermelon
	White flour (1/4 cup)
	White pepper
	Yogurt
	Zucchini squash
	Low/medium greens, beans and seeds:
	• Pumpkin seeds
	• Sunflower seeds
	• Kale, mustard greens, and collard greens (boiled)
	• Broccoli and Brussels sprouts (boiled)
	• Blackeyed peas, garbanzo beans, lima beans, mung beans, and red lentils
	Potato starch, chestnut flour, wild rice flour, coconut flour

Resources

The following list of resources is by no means comprehensive. It is meant simply to get you started on your further inquiry and research on some of the subject matter I present in this book. Like any curious researcher today, you must learn to Google your way to the information you seek. Recently, several autism organizations have affiliated around a common belief and intention – that autism is treatable, and recovery is possible. Autism.com is a great place to start.

It is my desire to create a comprehensive resource guide and community connection website that will serve as a research and implementation aid for all parents and practitioners exploring nutrition and dietary information. As this co-creation evolves, please feel free to contact me to participate.

Autism

Books

- *Changing the Course of Autism* by Bryan Jepson.
- *Healing the New Childhood Epidemics: Autism, ADHD, Asthma, and Allergies* by Kenneth Bock.
- *Autism, Brain and Environment* by Richard Lathe
- *Children with Starving Brains: A Medical Treatment Guide for Autism Spectrum Disorder* by Jaquelyn McCandless, MD
- *Biological Treatments for Autism and PDD* by Wlliam Shaw Ph.D.
- *Autism: Effective Biomedical Treatments (Have We Done Everything We Can For This Child? Individuality in an Epidemic)* by Jon Pangborn, Sidney Baker, and Bernard Rimland.
- *Louder Than Words: A Mother's Journey in Healing Autism* by Jenny McCarthy.
- *Mother Warriors,* by Jenny McCarthy

Websites

- Autism Research Institute: www.autism.com.
- DAN! Conference (Defeat Autism Now): www.danconference.com
- DAN! Webcast: www.autism.com/danwebcast
- Talk About Curing Autism Now (TACA): www.tacanow.com
- Cure Autism Now (CAN): www.cureautismnow.com
- Autism Speaks: http://www.autismspeaks.org
- Autism Society of America: www.autism-society.org
- National Autism Association: www.nationalautismassociation.org
- Generation Rescue: www.generationrescue.org
- Families for Early Autism Treatment: www.feat.org
- Unlocking Autism: www.unlockingautism.org
- Autism One: www.autismone.com
- Developmental Delay Resources: www.devdelay.org
- Autism Action Plan: www.AutismActionPlan.com
- DanasView.net
- Enzymestuff.com

Yahoo groups
- http://health.groups.yahoo.com/group/ANDI-ADI/
- http://health.groups.yahoo.com/group/EnzymesandAutism/
- http://health.groups.yahoo.com/group/DSI_Autism_PDD/
- http://health.groups.yahoo.com/group/chelatingkids2/
- http://health.groups.yahoo.com/group/Autism-Mercury/

Diets – Community Support
- Nourishing Hope for Autism Diet Community:
  http://www.facebook.com/group.php?gid=51745596033

Diets – Cooking and Recipes
- *Cooking to Heal* by Julie Matthews: CookingtoHeal.com
- gfcf-diet.talkaboutcuringautism.org/substitutions-gfcf-recipes.htm
- www.geocities.com/arnfl/diet.html - From Autism Recovery Network

Diets - GFCF
Books
- *Special Diets for Special Kids* by Lisa Lewis
- *Special Diets for Special Kids 2* by Lisa Lewis
- *Unraveling the Mystery of Autism* by Karen Seroussi
- *Gluten Free & Dairy Free Cooking* by Sueson Vess
- *The Kid-Friendly ADHD and Autism Cookbook* by Dana Laake and Pamela Compart

Websites
- www.gfcfdiet.com
- www.autismndi.com - Autism Network for Dietary Intervention
- www.celiac.com (gluten-free only, not casein-free)
- www.celiac.org (gluten-free)

Yahoo Groups
- http://health.groups.yahoo.com/group/GFCFKids/
- http://health.groups.yahoo.com/group/GFCFrecipes/
- http://groups.yahoo.com/group/FOODALLERGYKITCHEN/

Diets - SCD
Books
- *Breaking the Vicious Cycle: Intestinal Health Through Diet*, by Elaine Gottschall

Websites
- www.breakingthevicious cycle.info
- www.scdiet.com

- www.pecanbread.com
- www.lucyskitchenshop.com

Yahoo Groups
- http://health.groups.yahoo.com/group/ElainesChildren/
- http://health.groups.yahoo.com/group/pecanbread/
- http://health.groups.yahoo.com/group/SCDietkids/

Diets - Feingold Diet
- Why Can't My Child Behave? By Jane Hersey.
- www.feingold.org
- http://users.bigpond.net.au/allergydietitian/fi/salicylates-list.html - Full list of salicylate-levels in foods
- http://salicylatesensitivity.com
- http://salicylate-sensitivity.allergyanswers.net/

Diets- Low Oxalate Diet
- *The Low Oxalate Cookbook* available at the Vulvar Pain Foundation
  http://www.vulvarpainfoundation.org/vpfcookbook.htm
- VulvarPainFoundation.org – not autism specific but great research on oxalates
- http://health.groups.yahoo.com/group/Trying_Low_Oxalates/

Diets - Traditional Diets/Progressive Nutrition (raw dairy, fermented foods)
- *Nourishing Traditions* by Sally Fallon
- *The Fourfold Path to Healing*, by Thomas Cowan, MD
- Weston A. Price Foundation: www.WestonAPrice.org
- www.mercola.com - Dr. Joseph Mercola.
- www.realmilk.com
- http://health.groups.yahoo.com/group/FailsafeNT/
- http://health.groups.yahoo.com/group/lectins_in_autism/
- http://health.groups.yahoo.com/group/GFCFNN/

Diets - Yeast Diets
- *Body Ecology Diet*, by Donna Gates at www.bodyecologydiet.com
- *Feast Without Yeast*, By Bruce Semon
- *The Yeast Connection*, by William Crook

Food
- NuLife Foods – http://NuLifeFoods.com
- GFMeals.com
- www.EnjoyLifeFoods.com
- www.GlutenFree.com
- www.gluten.net (gluten-free)
- www.GlutenFreeda.com (Gourmet)

- www.GlutenFreeGourmet.com
- www.GlutenFreeMall.com (gluten-free)
- www.GlutenFreePantry.com
- www.ener-g.com
- www.AuthenticFoods.com - baking mixes
- www.PamelaProducts.com - cookies and mixes
- www.BreadsFromAnna.com
- www.CraveBakery.com

Vaccinations/Mercury Toxicity

- *What Your Doctor May Not Tell You About Vaccinations by Stephanie Cave, M.D.*
- *Evidence of Harm by David Kirby*
- *Amalgam Illness: Diagnosis and Treatment,* by Andrew Cutler
- *Hair Test Interpretation: Finding Hidden Toxicities*, by Andrew Cutler
- Vaccine Liberation Organization –exemptions forms and information, http://www.vaclib.org/exemption.htm
- http://www.gval.com/index.html - Global Vaccine Awareness League
- www.909shot.com - National Vaccine Information Center,
- www.generationrescue.org - Generation Rescue
- www.safeminds.org - Safe Minds

Food Allergies and Sensitivities

- *Is This Your Child? Discovering and Treating Unrecognized Allergies in Children and Adults* by Doris Rapp
- Bioset - http://www.bioset.net
- NAET - http://www.naet.com

Supplements/Products

- Brain Child Nutritionals: www.brainchildnutritionals.com
- Celtic Sea Salt: www.celticseasalt.com
- Custom Probiotics: www.customprobiotics.com
- GI ProHealth (GI ProStart Yogurt starter): www.giprohealth.com
- Himalayan Crystal Salt: www.americanbluegreen.com
- Houston Nutraceuticals: www.houstonni.com
- Kirkman: www.kirkmanlabs.com
- Klaire Labs: www.klaire.com
- New Beginnings Nutritionals: www.nbnus.com
- Nordic Naturals: www.nordicnaturals.com
- Nutricia (Neocate and EO28 Splash): www.nutricia.com/
- RevitaPop.com

Lab Assessments

- Doctor's Data: www.doctorsdata.com or (800) 323-2784
- Genova Diagnostics: www.gdx.net or (800) 522-4762
- Great Plains Laboratory: www.greatplainslaboratory.com or (913) 341-8949
- US Biotek: www.usbiotek.com or (206) 365-1256
- Metametrix Lab: www.metametrix.com
- Carbon Based Corporation: www.carbonbased.com
- ImmunoSciences Lab: www.immuno-sci-lab.com
- LEAP test (food and additive test): www.nowleap.com

Energy Medicine & Alternative Approaches

- *Anatomy of the Spirit,* by Caroline Myss
- *The Messages from Water,* by Masaru Emoto
- *Impossible Cure, by* Amy Lansky
- *Emotional Freedom Technique (EFT): www.emofree.com/*
- The Secret (Film – DVD): http://www.TheSecret.tv
- *What the Bleep Do We Know* (Film – DVD)
- Bioenergy Balancing - http://www.balancingcenter.com
- Cranial Sacral Therapy - http://www.craniosacraltherapy.org
- HANDLE Institute – www.handle.org

Environmentally-Friendly Products & Product Safety Cosmetics & Body Care

- Environmental Working Group report on cosmetics, safe and unsafe choices: http://ewg.org/reports/skindeep2/
- Fragrances and fragrance-free alternatives: http://www.nontoxic.com/nontoxic/fragrancefree.html
- Phthalates in cosmetics and body care: www.NotTooPretty.org

Products for a Safe Home and Healthy Child

- Children's Health Environmental Coalition: www.checnet.org
- Eco Design Resources: www.ecodesignresources.com
- Green Fusion Design Center: www.greenfusiondesigncenter.com
- Green Home- Great resource for natural apparel, toys, bedding at: www.greenhome.com
- Happy Planet - "Organic fibers for everyday and every night: www.ahappyplanet.com
- NonToxic - Organic mattresses, bedding, and healthy home products: http://www.nontoxic.com

Health and Environmental News and Product Reports

- Bioneers - Visionary and practical solutions for restoring the Earth at: http://www.bioneers.org/
- Environmental Health News - news and information at: www.environmentalhealthnews.org
- Environmental Working Group at: http://ewg.org
- The Green Guide at: www.TheGreenGuide.com
- www.Mindfully.org
- www.SustainLane.com

BIBLIOGRAPHY

Adams JB, "Summary of Biomedical Treatments for Autism," ARI Publication 40 / April 2007

Adams JB, et al. Abnormally high plasma levels of vitamin B6 in children with autism not taking supplements compared to controls not taking supplements. *The Journal of Alternative and Complementary Medicine* - 01-JAN-2006; 12(1): 59-63

Adams JB, George F, Audhya T. Abnormally high plasma levels of vitamin B6 in children with autism not taking supplements compared to controls not taking supplements. J Altern Complement Med. 2006 Jan-Feb;12(1):59-63. .

Adams JB, Holloway C. Pilot Study of a Moderate Dose Multivitamin/Mineral Supplement for Children with Autistic Spectrum Disorder. *The Journal of Alternative and Complementary Medicine.* 2004, 10(6): 1033-1039. doi:10.1089/acm.2004.10.1033.

Alberti, A., Pirrone, P., Elia, M., Waring, R.H. & Romano, C., "Sulphation deficit in low-functioning autistic children: a pilot study." *Biological Psychiatry*, 46, 420-424.

Allen, G., et al. "Phosphatase as a measure of pasteurization." *Commun Dis Public Health*, 2004, Jun;7(2):96-101.

Article and updates available at: http://autism.asu.edu.

Baird G, Simonoff E, Pickles A, Chandler S, Loucas T, Meldrum D, Charman T. Prevalence of disorders of the autism spectrum in a population cohort of children in South Thames: the Special Needs and Autism Project (SNAP). *Lancet.* 2006 Jul 15;368(9531):210-5.

Bauman, M., and Kemper, T., *The Neurobiology of Autism.* The John Hopkins University Press, Baltimore, MD, 1994.

Ben-Menachem E. "Nonpharmacologic Treatments of Epilepsy." American Epilepsy Society 58th Annual Meeting; December 3-7, 2004; New Orleans, Louisiana.

Berglund F. Improved Health After Removal Of Dental Amalgam Fillings. Analysis Of Studies Published 1986-1997. http://www.tf.nu/artiklar/fakta_berglund_forb_halsa_analys_studier_1986-1997_eng.shtml

Bernard, S., Enayati, A., Redwood, L., Roger, H., Binstock, T., "Autism: A Novel Form of Mercury Poisoning." *Medical Hypotheses* (2001) 56(4), 462-71.

Bertrand J, Mars A, Boyle C, Bove F, Yeargin-Allsopp M, Decoufle P. Prevalence of autism in a United States population: the Brick Township, New Jersey, investigation.

Bishayi B, Sengupta M. Synergism in immunotoxicological effects due to repeated combined administration of arsenic and lead in mice. *Int Immunopharmacol.* 2006 Mar;6(3):454-64.

Björnberg KA, Vahter M, Petersson-Grawé K, Glynn A, Cnattingius S, Darnerud PO, Atuma S, Aune M, Becker W, Berglund M. Methyl mercury and inorganic mercury in Swedish pregnant women and in cord blood: influence of fish consumption. *Environ Health Perspect.* 2003 Apr;111(4):637-41

Block, MA, www.blockcenter.com/autism.htm

Blum K, Sheridan PJ, Wood RC, Braverman ER, Chen TJ, Cull JG, Comings DE. The D2 dopamine receptor gene as a determinant of reward deficiency syndrome. : *J R Soc Med.* 1996 Jul;89(7):396-400.

Bock, Kenneth, *Healing the New Childhood Epidemics: Autism, ADHD, Asthma, and Allergies.* Ballantine Books, New York, NY, 2007.

Boyd E. Haley, PhD and Teri Small. Interview with Dr. Boyd E. Haley: Biomarkers supporting mercury toxicity as the major exacerbator of neurological illness, recent evidence via the urinary porphyrin tests

Medical Veritas 3 (2006) 921–934 921 (interview on Autism One Radio).
http://www.whale.to/v/haley.pdf

Brain/Mind Bulletin, "Life Energy Patterns Visible Via New Technique," vol. 7, no. 14 (August 23) 1982.

Braverman, E. Pfeiffer, C. *The Healing Nutrients Within*. Keats Publishing, New Canaan , Connecticut. 1987. pgs 191-210

Breitkreutz R, Pittack N, Nebe CT, Schuster D, Brust J, Beichert M, Hack V, Daniel V, Edler L, Droge W. Improvement of immune functions in HIV infection by sulfur supplementation: two randomized trials. *J Mol Med*. 2000;78(1):55-62.

Brimacombe M, Xue Ming , Parikh A. Familial risk factors in autism. *J Child Neurol*. 2007 May;22(5):593-7.

Brown, M.J., Ferruzzi M.G. et al. "Carotenoid Bioavailability is Higher from Salads Ingested with Full-Fat than with Fat-Reduced Salad Dressing as measure with Electrochemical Detection." *American Journal of Clinical Nutrition*, 2004;80:396-403.

Bryd, Robert. MIND Institute. Report to the Legislature on the Principle Findings from the Epidemiology of Autism in California: A Comprehensive Pilot Study. UC Davis 17 October 2002. http://www.dds.ca.gov/autism/pdf/study_final.pdf

Campos FA, Flores H, Underwood BA. Effect of an infection on vitamin A status of children as measured by the relative dose response (RDR). Am J Clin Nutr. 1987 Jul;46(1):91-4.

Carroll, Lee and Tober, Jan, *The Indigo Children*. Hay House, Inc. Carlsbad, CA, 1999.

Cave, Stephanie. *What Your Doctor May Not Tell You About Children's Vaccinations*. Warner Books, Inc. New York, NY, 2001.

CDC: Autism A.L.A.R.M January 2004
http://www.medicalhomeinfo.org/health/autism%20downloads/autismalarm.pdf

Chowdhury S, Kumar R, Ganguly NK, Kumar L, Walia BN. Effect of vitamin A supplementation on childhood morbidity and mortality. Indian J Med Sci. 2002 Jun;56(6):259-64

Cockell KA, Bonacci G, Belonje B. Manganese content of soy or rice beverages is high in comparison to infant formulas. J Am Coll Nutr. 2004 Apr;23(2):124-30.

Cohen et al. "Pica and Elevated Blood Lead Level in Autistic and Atypical Children." *American Journal of Disabled Children*, Vol. 130, January 1976.

Comi, A.M., Zimmerman, A.W., Frye, V.H., Law, P.A., Peeden, J.N. "Familial Clustering of Autoimmune Disorders and Evaluation of Medical Risk Factors in Autism." *Journal of Child Neurology*, 1999, June,14 (6):388-94.

Comings DE. Clinical and molecular genetics of ADHD and Tourette syndrome. Two related polygenic disorders. Ann N Y Acad Sci. 2001 Jun;931:50-83.

Crook, W., *The Yeast Connection: A Medical Breakthrough*. Random House, New York, NY, 1986.

Cummins, Ronnie & Ben Lilliston, Genetically Engineered Food, Herlowe & Co., NY, 2000.

Cutler, Andrew, Amalgam Illness, Diagnosis and Treatment: What You Can Do to Get Better, How Your Doctor Can Help. Sammamish, WA, 1999.

Cutler, Andrew, Hair Test Interpretation: Finding Hidden Toxicities. 2004.

DAN syllabus, Seattle Washington, Fall 2006,

DeFelice, Karen. *Enzymes: Go With Your Gut*. ThunderSnow Interactive, Minnesota, 2006.

DeFelice, Karen. *Enzymes For Autism and other Neurological Conditions*. ThunderSnow Interactive, Minnesota, 2003.

Deluca HF, Cantorna MT. Vitamin D: its role and uses in immunology. *The FASEB Journal*. 2001;15:2579-258.

Department of Developmental Services, *A Report to the Legislature; Changes in the Population of Persons with Autism and Pervasive Developmental Disorders in California's Developmental Services System: 1987 through 1998*. Sacramento, CA, March 1, 1999.

Deth, Richard C., *Molecular Aspects of Thimerisol-Induced Autism*, Committee on Government Reform Testimony, Boston, MA

Di Cagno, R., et al. "Sourdough Bread Made from Wheat and Nontoxic Flours and Started with Selected Lactobacilli is Tolerated in Celiac Sprue Patients." *Applied and Environmental Microbiology*, Feb. 2004, p.1088-1096.

Donnelly S, Loscher CE, Lynch MA, and Mills KH. "Whole-cell but not acellular pertussis vaccines induce convulsive activity in mice: evidence of a role for toxin-induced interleukin-1beta in a new murine model for analysis of neuronal side effects of vaccination." *Infect Immun* - 2001; 69(7): 4217-23

Environmental Working Group: A benchmark investigation of industrial chemicals, pollutants and pesticides in umbilical cord blood. July 14, 2005 http://archive.ewg.org/reports/bodyburden2/execsumm.php

Fallon, Sally. Nourishing Traditions. New Trends Publishing, Washington D.C., 2001.

Faraone, S., and Biederman, J., "Do Attention Deficit Hyperactivity Disorder and Major Depression Share Familial Risk Factors?" *Journal of Nervous and Mental Disease*, 185 (9) September, 1997: 533-41.

Fombonne E, Zakarian R, Bennett A, Meng L, McLean-Heywood D. Pervasive developmental disorders in Montreal, Quebec, Canada: prevalence and links with immunizations. *Pediatrics*. 2006 Jul;118(1):e139-50.

Fudenberg, H. Dialysable lymphocyte extract (DLyE) in infantile onset autism: a pilot study. *Biotherapy* 19:144, 1996

Garland CF, Garland FC, Gorham ED, Lipkin M, Newmark H, Mohr SB, Holick MF. The role of vitamin D in cancer prevention. Am J Public Health. 2006 Feb;96(2):252-61.

Geier DA, Geier MR. A case series of children with apparent mercury toxic encephalopathies manifesting with clinical symptoms of regressive autistic disorders. *J Toxicol Environ Health A*. 2007 May 15;70(10):837-51.

Geier DA, Geier MR. A clinical and laboratory evaluation of methionine sycle-transsulfuration and androgen pathway markers in children with autistic disorders. Hormone Research. 2006:66(4):182-8. Epub 2006 Jul 5.

Geier DA, Geier MR. A prospective study of thimerosal-containing Rho(D)-immune globulin administration as a risk factor for autistic disorders. *J Matern Fetal Neonatal Med*. 2007 May;20 (5):385-90.

Gillberg C, Cederlund M, Lamberg K, Zeijlon L. Brief report: "the autism epidemic." The registered prevalence of autism in a Swedish urban area. *J Autism Dev Disord*. 2006 Apr;36(3):429-35.

Gilliland, F.D., et al., "Maternal and Grandmaternal Smoking Patterns Are Associated With Early Childhood Asthma." *Chest*. 2005;127:1232-1241.

Golub MS, Hogrefe CE, Germann SL, Tran TT, Beard JL, Crinella FM, Lonnerdal B Neurobehavioral evaluation of rhesus monkey infants fed cow's milk formula, soy formula, or soy formula with added manganese. *Neurotoxicol Teratol*. 2005 Jul-Aug;27(4):615-27.

Gottschall, Elaine. *Breaking the Vicious Cycle*. The Kirkton Press, Baltimore, Ontario, Canada, 2002.

Grant WB, Garland CF, Gorham ED. An estimate of cancer mortality rate reductions in Europe and the US with 1,000 IU of oral vitamin D per day.

Greenwalt, C.J., Ledford, R.A., Steinkraus, K.A., *Kombucha Mushroom Tea, Is it Safe? Determination and characterization of the anti-microbial activity of the fermented tea Kombucha*. C.J. Department of Food Science Cornell University Ithaca, New York, 1998.

Gupta C. Reproductive Malformation of the Male Offspring Following Maternal Exposure to Estrogenic Chemicals. Proceedings of the Society for Experimental Biology and Medicine 224:61-68 Jun00

Gupta, S., et al., "Th1- and Th2-like cytokines in CD4+ and CD8+ T-cells in Autism." *Journal of Neuroimmunology* 85 (1998) 106-109.

Haley, B. Testimony Before the House Government Reform Committee. November 14, 2002. http://www.whale.to/vaccine/hayley.html

Heafield, M, *et al.*, "Plasma cysteine and sulphate levels in patients with motor neuron, Parkinson's and Alzheimer's disease." *Neuroscience Letters*, 110:216-220, 1990.

Health Canada: The Safety of Dental Amalgam 1996 http://www.hc-sc.gc.ca/dhp-mps/alt_formats/hpfb-dgpsa/pdf/md-im/dent_amalgam_e.pdf

Hendel, Barbara and Ferreira, Peter. *Water & Salt, The Essence of Life*. Natural Resources, 2003.

Hersey, Jane. *Why Can't My Child Behave?* Pear Tree Press, Inc. Alexandria, VA, 2002.

Hickenbottom, S.J., Follett, J.R., Lin Y., Dueker, S.R., Burri, B.J., Neidlinger, T.R. and Clifford, A.J. "Variability in Conversion of Beta-Carotene to vitamin A in Men as Measured by using a Double-Tracer Study Design." *American Journal of Clinical Nutrition*, 2002;75:900-7.

Hobeisen, D.F., et al., "Grass fed cows and omega-3 in milk." *International Journal for Vitamin and Nutrition Research*, 1993;63(3):229-33.

Holick MF. Sunlight and vitamin D for bone health and prevention of autoimmune diseases, cancers, and cardiovascular disease. Am J Clin Nutr. 2004 Dec;80(6 Suppl):1678S-88S.

Homiston, S., and Good, C., *Vaccinating Your Child: Questions and Answers for the Concerned Parent*, Peachtree Publishers, Atlanta, GA, 2000.

Hsu CS, Liu PL, Chien LC, Chou SY, Han BC Mercury concentration and fish consumption in Taiwanese pregnant women. BJOG. 2007 Jan;114(1):81-5.

http://homeopathy-cures.com, Classic Homeopathy, Inc.

http://www.atsdr.cdc.gov/toxprofiles/tp46.html#bookmark11

Icasiano F, Hewson P, Machet P, Cooper C, Marshall A. Childhood autism spectrum disorder in the Barwon region: a community based study. *J Paediatr Child Health*. 2004 Dec;40(12):696-701.

Isolauri, E. Probiotics in human disease. *American Journal of Clinical Nutrition*, Vol. 73, No. 6, 1142S-1146S, June 2001

James SJ, Cutler P, Melnyk S, Jernigan S, Janak L, Gaylor DW, Neubrander JA. Metabolic biomarkers of increased oxidative stress and impaired methylation capacity in children with autism. American Journal of Clinical Nutrition. 2004 Dec;80(6):1611-7.

James SJ, Melnyk S, Jernigan S, Cleves MA, Halsted CH, Wong DH, Cutler P, Bock K, Boris M, Bradstreet JJ, Baker SM, Gaylor DW. Metabolic endophenotype and related genotypes are associated with oxidative stress in children with autism. American Journal of Medical Genetics, Part B: Neuropsychiatric Genetics. 2006 Dec 5:141(8):947-56

James, J et al. "Abnormal Levels of Transsulfuration and methionine cycle metabolic intermediates in autism indicate impaired redox status." *J Clin Invest*. Manuscript under review.

Jepson, Bryan. *Changing the Course of Autism*. Sentient Publications, Boulder, Colorado, 2007.

Johnston et al, Vitamin C elevates red blood cell glutathione in healthy adults. Am J Clin Nutr. 1993 Jul;58(1):103-5.

Kaufmann WE, Cortell R, Kau AS, Bukelis I, Tierney E, Gray RM, Cox C, Capone GT, Stanard P. Autism spectrum disorder in fragile X syndrome: communication, social interaction, and specific behaviors. *Am J Med Genet A*. 2004 Sep 1;129(3):225-34.

Kawashima H, et al. "Detection and sequencing of measles virus from peripheral mononuclear cells from patients with inflammatory bowel disease and autism." *Dig Dis Sci*. 2000, Apr;45(4):723-9.

Kenmoku H., et al, "Erinacine C, a new erinacine from Hericium erinaceus, and its biosynthetic route to erinancine C in the basidiomycete." *Bioscience Biotechnology Biochemistry*, 2002, Mar;66(3):571-75.

Kilburn, K.H. "Exposure to Reduced Sulfur Gases Impairs Neurobehavioral Function." *Southern Medical Journal*, 90:10, 997-1006, 1997.

Kirby, David. *Evidence of Harm*. St. Martin's Press, New York, NY, 2005.

Knell ER, Comings DE. Tourette's syndrome and attention-deficit hyperactivity disorder: evidence for a genetic relationship. *J Clin Psychiatry*. 1993 Sep;54(9):331-7.

Krauss, W.E., Erb, J.H. and Washburn, R.G. Studies on the nutritive value of milk, II. "The effect of pasteurization on some of the nutritive properties of milk," *Ohio Agricultural Experiment Station Bulletin* 518, page 9, January, 1933.

Lang, M. Conversations, 2002.

Lang, Michael, "Autism and Potential Causal Factors: Towards a Unified Theoretical Model." Published: www.brainchildnutritionals.com, 2000.

Langford, Willis. "Comprehensive Guide to Managing Autism," Revised August 2001. Downloaded at: http://www.vaccinationnews.com/DailyNews/August2001/CompGuideManageAut.htm

Lansky, Amy. Impossible Cure: The Promise of Homeopathy. R.L. Ranch Press, Portola Valley, CA, 2003.

Lee, Lita, Turner, Lisa, and Goldberg, Burton. The Enzyme Cure. AlternativeMedicine.com Books, Tiburon, CA, 1998.

Leitzmann, Et al, *Dietary intake of n–3 and n–6 fatty acids and the risk of prostate cancer,* American Journal of Clinical Nutrition, Vol. 80, No. 1, 204-216, July 2004.

Ley, B., Immune System Control: Colostrum and Lactoferrin. BL Publications, Detroit Lakes, MN, 2000.

Lingam R, Simmons A, Andrews N, Miller E, Stowe J, Taylor B. Prevalence of autism and parentally reported triggers in a north east London population. Archives of Disease in Childhood. 88:666-670. 2003.

Loscher, CE, Donnelly S, Lynch MA and Mills KH. "Induction of inflammatory cytokines in the brain following respiratory infection with Bordetella pertussis." *J. Neuroimmunol*. 2000; 102(2): 172-81

Lotspeich, L.J. and Ciaranello, R.D., "The Neurobiology and Genetics of Infantile Autism." *International Review of Neurobiology*, Vol. 35, 87-122, 1993.

Lynch, Laurie, ND, PhD candidate-Nutrition, *The Health Hazards of Genetically Engineering Foods* http://www.biowatch.org.za/docs/health_hazards.pdf

Marques RC, Dórea JG, Fonseca MF, Bastos WR, Malm O. Eur J Pediatr. Hair mercury in breast-fed infants exposed to thimerosal-preserved vaccines. 2007 Sep;166(9):935-41.

Martineau, J., Barthelemy, C., Garreau, B., Lelord, G. "Vitamin b6, Magnesium and combined B6-Mg Therapteutic Effects in Childhood Autism." *Biol Psychiatry*, 1985;20:467-478.

Mathews Larson, J. Depression-Free Naturally. (New York, Random House, 1999).

McCandless, J., *Children with Starving Brains*. Bramble Books, Canada, 2004.

McCormick LH. Depression in mothers of children with attention deficit hyperactivity disorder. Fam Med. 1995 Mar;27(3):176-9.

McCraty, R. "Modulation of DNA Conformation by Heart-Focused Intention." HeartMath Research Center, Institute of HeartMath, Publication No. 03-008. Boulder Creek, CA, 2003.

Megson, MN "Is Autism a G-Alpha Protein Defect Reversible with Natural Vitamin A?" *Medical Hypotheses*, 2000, June;54(6):979-83, downloaded from www.megson.com/hypothesis/medical_hypothesis_article.html, p 1-6.

Megson, MN. Presentation at the DAN! Conference on "Is Autism a G-Alpha ProteinDefect Reversible with Natural Vitamin A?" 1999.

Mercola.com, Dr. Joseph Mercola's Website

Mosby's Medical Dictionary, *Mosby, Inc*. St. Louis, Missouri, 2002.

Mouridsen SE, Rich B, Isager T, Nedergaard NJ. Autoimmune diseases in parents of children with infantile autism: a case-control study. Dev Med Child Neurol. 2007 Jun;49(6):429-32.

Moynahan, E.J., "Zinc Deficiency and Disturbances of Mood and Behavior." *Lancet*, Jan 10;1(7950):91, 1976.

Murch, S.H., MacDonald, T.T., Walker-Smith, J.A., Levin, M., Lionetti, P., & Klein, N.J. "Disruption of Sulphated Glucosaminoglycans in Intestinal Inflammation." *Lancet*, 341, 711-714, 1993.

Murray, M., *Encyclopedia of Nutritional Supplements*. Prima Publishing, Rocklin, CA, 1996.

Nofech-Mozes Y, et al. "Induction of mRNA for tumor necrosis factor-alpha and interleukin-1 beta in mice brain, spleen and liver in an animal model of Shigella-related seizures." *Isr. Med. Assoc. J.* 2000:2,86-90.

Null, G. *The Food-Mood-Body Connection*. Seven Stories Press, New York, NY, 2000.

NY Times, "Increase in Autism Baffles Scientists" by Sandra Blakeslee, October 18, 2002.

Ohio EPA. "Antimony and Antimony Compounds." Pollution Prevention Factsheet. Number 102. September 2002. http://www.epa.state.oh.us/opp/mercury_pbt/fact102.pdf

Ou S, Gao K, and Li Y. An in Vitro Study of Wheat Bran Binding Capacity for Hg, Cd, and Pb. *J. Agric. Food Chem.*, 47 (11), 4714 -4717, 1999.

Owens, S.C. "Explorations of the new Frontier Between Gut and Brain:A Look at GAGs, CCK, and motilin." *Psychobiology of Autism: Current Research and Practice*. Van Mildert College, University of Durham, April 15-17th, 45-70, 1998. Copy emailed by Owens p. 1-22.

Owens, S.C. "Sulfate Regulation and its Neurodevelopmental Role." *Proceedings of an Autism Odyssey.* Van Mildert College, University of Durham, April 5th, 217-235, 2001. Copy emailed by Owens p. 1-24.

Pangborn, J. and Baker, S. *Biomedical Assessment Options for Children with Autism and Related Problems.* Autism Research Institute, San Diego, CA, 2002.

Pediatrics. 2001 Nov;108(5):1155-61.

Peterson JD, Herzenberg LA, Vasquez K, Waltenbaugh C. "Glutathione levels in antigen-presenting cells modulate Th1 versus Th2 response patterns." *Proc Nat Acad Sci USA* 1998;95: 3071-3076.

Pfeiffer, C. Nutrition and Mental Illness: An Orthomolecular Approach to Balancing Body Chemistry

Pizzorno, Joseph, *Total Wellness.* Prima Health, Rocklin, CA, 1998, p. 94-106.

Ponnampalam, E.N., Mann, N.J., Sinclair, A.J. "Effect of Feeding Systems on Omega-3 Fatty acids, Conjugated Linoleic Acid and Trans Fatty Acids in Australian Beef Cuts: Potential Impact on Human Health." *Asia Pac J. Clin Nutr.* 2006;15(1):21-9.

Powers, M., *Children with Autism: A Parents' Guide.* Woodbine House, Bethesda, MD, 2000.

Rapp, D., *Is this Your Child? Discovering and Treating Unrecognized Allergies in Children and Adults.* William Morrow and Company, New York, NY, 1991.

Reichelt KL, Knivsberg AM. Can the pathophysiology of autism be explained by the nature of the discovered urine peptides? *Nutr Neurosci.* 2003 Feb;6(1):19-28

Richard, Lathe. *Autism, Brain, and Environment.* Jessica Kingsley Publishers. Philidelphia, PA, 2006.

Rimland B, Callaway E, Dreyfus P. The effect of high doses of vitamin B6 on autistic children: a double-blind crossover study. Am J Psychiatry. 1978 Apr;135(4):472-5.

Rimland, B. High dosage levels of certain vitamins in the treatment of children with severe mental disorders.In D. Hawkins & L. Pauling (Eds.), *Orthomolecular Psychiatry.* New York: W.H. Freeman, (pp. 513-538), 1973.

Rimland, B., " Controversies in the Treatment of Autistic Children: Vitamin and Drug Therapy." *Journal of Child Neurology*, Vol. 3, Supplement, 1988, p. S68-S71.

Risch, N, et. al. A Genomic Screen of Autism: Evidence for a Multilocus Etiology. *Am. J. Hum. Genet.,* 65:493-507, 1999.

Rogers, Sherry. *Detoxify or Die.* Sand Key Company, Sarasota, FL, 2002.

Rooney JPK. The role of thiols, dithiols, nutritional factors and interacting ligands in the toxicology of mercury. *Toxicology.* Volume 234, Issue 3, 20 May 2007, Pages 145-156

Ross, J. The Mood Cure. (New York, Penguin, 2002}

Rule, D.C., Broughton, K.S., Shellito, S.M., Maiorano G. "Comparison of Muscle Fatty Acid Profiles and Cholesterol Concentrations of Bison, Beef Cattle, Elk, and Chicken." *Journal of Animal Science.* 2002. 80:1202-1211.

Safe Harbor – International Guide to the World of Alternative Mental Health – Pyroluria, May 2004 http://www.alternativementalhealth.com/articles/pyroluria.htm

Schauss, Mark. Conversation. 2006.

Schubert J, Riley EJ, Tyler SA. Combined effects in toxicology--a rapid systematic testing procedure: cadmium, mercury, and lead. J Toxicol Environ Health. 1978 Sep-Nov;4(5-6):763-76.

Shattock Paul and Whiteley, Paul, *An increasing incidence of autism*? University of Sunderland, UK, 2001.

Shaw, W. *Biological Treatments for Autism and PDD*, William Shaw, Overland Park, KS, 1998.

Shcherbatykh I, Carpenter DO. The role of metals in the etiology of Alzheimer's disease. JAlzheimers Dis. 2007 May;11(2):191-205.

Shift Magazine: Dec 2004 – Feb 2005

Sinzig JK, Lehmkuhl G. Autism and ADHD - are there common traits? Fortschr Neurol Psychiatr. 2007 May;75(5):267-74.

Stoll, A., The Omega-3 Connection. Simon & Schuster, New York, NY, 2001.

Strunecka, Anna, Patocka, Jiri, Schuld, Andreas, AlFx: the useful tool in laboratory investigations, but potential danger for humans. Department of Physiology and Developmental Biology, Czech Republic.

Sunlight. *Recent Results Cancer Res.* 2007;174:225-34.

The Secret (DVD)

Thurnham DI, Northrop-Clewes CA, McCullough FSW, Das BS, Lunn, PG. Innate Immunity, Gut Integrity, and Vitamin A in Gambian and Indian Infants. *The Journal of Infectious Diseases.* 2000; 182(Suppl 1):S23–8.

Tilgner, S., *Herbal Medicine From the Heart of the Earth.* Wise Acres Press, Creswell, OR, 1999.

U.S. Department of Health and Human Services and U.S. Environmental Protection Agency. Mercury Levels in Commercial Fish and Shellfish. February 2006. http://www.cfsan.fda.gov/~frf/sea-mehg.html

Vargas, D.L., Nascimbene, C., Krishnan, C., Zimmerman, A.W., Pardo, C.A. "Neuroglial Activation and Neuroinflammation in the Brain of Patients with Autism." *Annals of Neurology*; Feb;57(2):304, 2005

Veenstra-VanDerWeele, J, Cook EH. Genetics of Childhood Disorders:XLVI. Autism, Part 5: Genetics of Autism. *J Am Acad Child Adolesc Psychiatry*,42:1,116-118 January 2003

Virture, Doreen. The Care and Feeding of Indigo Children. Hay House, Inc., Carlsbad, CA, 2001.

Wakefield AJ, et al. "Detection and Sequencing of Measles Virus from Peripheral Mononuclear Cells from Patients with Inflammatory Bowel Disease and Autism." *Digestive Diseases and Sciences*, Vol. 45, No. 4: 723-729, April 2000.

Wakefield AJ, et al., "Potential Viral Pathogenic mechanism for New Variant Inflammatory Bowel Disease." *Mol Pathol*, 2002, Apr:55(2):84-90.

Waring R.H. et al. "Metabolism of low-dose paracetamol in patients with rheumatoid arthritis." *Xenobiotica*, Vol. 21, No. 5:689-693, 1991.

Waring R.H., and Klovrza, L.V. "Sulphur Metabolism in Autism." *Journal of Nutritional and Evironmental Medicine*, 10,25-32.

Waring, R.H. Ngong, J.M., Klovrza, L.V. Green, S., & Sharp, H. "Biochemical Parameters in Autistic Children." *Developmental Brain Dysfunnction*, 10, 40-43.

Waring, R.H., & O'Reilly, B.A. "Enzyme and sulphur ozidation Deficiences in Autistic Children with Known Food/Chemical Intolerances." *Xenobiotica*, 20, 117-122.

Waser, M., et. al., "Inverse association of farm milk consumption with asthma and allergy in rural and suburban populations across Europe." *Clinical and Experimental Allergy*, Dec, 20, 2006.

Waterland RA, Dolinoy DC, Lin JR, Smith CA, Shi X, Tahiliani KG. Maternal methyl supplements increase offspring DNA methylation at Axin Fused. *Genesis*. 2006 Sep;44(9):401-6.

Waterland RA, Jirtle RL. Early nutrition, epigenetic changes at transposons and imprinted genes, and enhanced susceptibility to adult chronic diseases. *Nutrition*. 2004 Jan;20(1):63-8

Waterland RA, Jirtle RL. Transposable elements: targets for early nutritional effects on epigenetic gene regulation. *Mol Cell Biol*. 2003 Aug;23(15):5293-300.

Waterland RA. Assessing the Effects of High Methionine Intake on DNA Methylation.. *The American Society for Nutrition J. Nutr*. 136:1706S-1710S, June 2006.

Wecker et al. "Trace Element Concentrations in Hair From Autistic Children." *Journal Ment. Defic. Res*. 29:15-22, 1985.

What the @%&# (Bleep) Do We Know? (DVD)

William J. Walsh, Anjum Usman, and Jeffrey Tarpey. Disordered Metal Metabolism in a Large Autism Population. Findings presented at the American Psychiatric Association 2001 Annual Meeting (New Orleans, LA, May 5-10, 2001), and at the International Meeting for Autism Research (San Diego, CA, November 10, 2001). Health Research Institute and Pfeiffer Treatment Center http://hriptc.org/metal_autism.html

Woo EJ, Ball R, Landa R, Zimmerman AW, Braun MM . Developmental regression and autism reported to the Vaccine Adverse Event Reporting System. Autism. 2007 Jul;11(4):301-10. }

Xue F, Holzman C, Rahbar MH, Trosko K, Fischer L. Maternal fish consumption, mercury levels, and risk of preterm delivery. *Environ Health Perspect*. 2007 Jan;115(1):42-7.

Yeargin-Allsopp M, Rice C, Karapurkar T, Doernberg N, Boyle C, Murphy C. Prevalence of autism in a US metropolitan area. *JAMA*. 2003 Jan 1;289(1):49-55

Young, R.O., *Sick and Tired?* Woodland Publishing, Pleasant Grove, UT, 1999.

Zand, J, et al., *Smart Medicine for a Healthier Child*. Penguin Putnam, New York, NY, 1994.

Zapata-Sirvent, R.L., Hansbrough, J.F., Greenleaf, G.E., Grayson, L.S., Wolf, P. "Reduction of Bacterial Translocation and of Intestinal Structural Alterations By Heparin in a Murine Burn Injury Model." *Journal of Trauma*. 36, 1-6, 1994.

Zimmerman, M., *A.D.D. Nutrition Solution: A Drug-Free 30-Day Plan*. Henry Holt and Company, New York, NY, 1999.

Zitterman A, Effects of Vitamin K on calcium and bone metabolism, Curr Opin Clin Nutr Metab Care, 2001 Nov;4(6):483-7.

Index

5

5-HTP, 91

A

Acetic Acid, 151
Acetaminophen, 17
ADHD, 17, 18, 42, 47, 116, 117
Adrenal extract or glandular, 92
Adrenals, 93
Agouti mice, 13
Allergenic Foods, 138
Aluminum, 26, 32, 121, 126
Amalgam, 19, 22, 23, 24, 125
Amine, 47, 105, 117, 150, 198
Amino acids, 22, 35, 40, 43, 48, 50, 60, 65, 80, 81, 82, 85, 88, 151, 158, 161
Amygdala, 173
Antibiotics, 11, 32, 34, 74, 87, 119, 177, 188, 189, 190
Antibodies, 27, 30, 32, 34, 40, 151, 176, 179
Antibody blood test, 139
Anti-inflammatory, 84, 131, 145
Antioxidants, 43, 44, 50, 53, 70, 71, 72, 79, 92, 93, 196
Arginine, 145
Arm flapping, 20, 172
Artificial Ingredients/Food Additives, 116
Artificial Sweeteners, 118
Ashwaganda, 92
Aspartate, 118
Assessments, 66
Asthma, 55, 94, 98, 105
Astragalus Root, 93
Autoimmune, 17, 18, 27, 28, 44, 54, 55, 172, 173
Autoimmune disease, 22
Autoimmune disorder, 16, 17, 18
Autoimmune reaction, 28, 30, 36, 50, 75, 147

B

B12, 42, 64, 74, 91, 151, 161
B6, 64, 72, 73, 143, 151, 158, 161, 200, 201, 215
Baker, Sidney, 73, 113, 175
Beans, 143
Bernard, Sallie, 20, 172, 174
bicarbonate, 50, 51, 61, 156
Bile salts, 51, 202
Biochemical imbalances, 5, 169
biochemistry, 51, 54, 68, 69
Bioenergy Balancing, 91
Biomedical, 187
Biotin, 64, 74, 156, 158
Blackstrap molasses, 143, 146
Bloating, 33, 85, 118, 202
Body Ecology Diet, 95, 100, 101, 107, 149, 152, 207
Brainchild Nutritionals, 92, 157, 186
Breathing, 61
Broccoli, 49, 76, 79, 91, 105, 108, 111, 161
Broths, 144

Burdock Root, 93
Butyric acid, 61, 88, 151, 157

C

Cabbage, 76, 91, 161
Calcium, 27, 49, 61, 79, 91, 143, 144, 174, 181
Calcium oxalate, 200
Calcium, non-dairy sources, 79
Calories, 129
Candida, 32, 33, 34, 44, 88, 89, 100, 101, 107, 150, 151, 155, 156, 161, 186
Carbohydrates, 46, 50, 133
Carnitine, 81
Casein, 22, 30, 35, 36, 44, 48, 85, 95, 97, 98, 99, 128, 136, 149, 179, 192, 206
Caseomorphins, 85
Cave, Stephanie, 28, 29, 30, 31, 175, 208
CBS, 14, 132
CCK, 46, 51
Celiac, 100, 206
Chelation, 78, 79, 113, 164
Chlorine, 47, 122, 184
Cholesterol, 131, 132
Chromium, 118
CO2, 60, 61
Coconut oil, 131
Cod liver oil, 32, 55, 71, 75, 83, 127, 175
Coenzyme, 90
Colostrum, 88, 158
Comi, Ann, 17, 18
Constipation, 33, 35, 36, 85, 96, 97, 98, 102, 106, 138, 150, 172
Corn, 35
Crohn's disease, 29, 30
Cysteine, 40, 43, 44, 45, 49, 77, 80, 82, 158, 161
Cytokines, 11

D

Dairy, 30, 33, 35, 66, 75, 79, 97, 99, 100, 103, 116, 119, 135, 149, 157, 179
Dairy, raw, 99, 149, 187, 191, 207
DAN, 9, 20, 34, 44, 52, 69, 70, 72, 79, 80, 94, 95, 156
Depression, 18, 35, 93, 102
Detoxification, 17, 22, 26, 37, 43, 44, 45, 46, 48, 49, 53, 54, 67, 77, 79, 90, 92, 94, 113, 117, 119, 122, 140, 150, 151, 158, 161, 162, 164, 184
DHA, 79, 83, 158
DHEA, 46, 159
Diarrhea, 33, 35, 36, 61, 72, 74, 77, 78, 85, 88, 94, 95, 96, 97, 98, 100, 104, 106, 118, 138, 157, 165, 172, 202
Digestion, 11, 37, 45, 46, 50, 51, 56, 66, 73, 83, 85, 90, 93, 97, 150, 151, 154, 155
Dipeptidyl dipeptidase, 85
DMAE, 91
DMG, 59, 77, 80
DMSA, 113
DNA, 33, 40, 74, 119
DNA Methylation, DNA, 15

Down syndrome, 15, 43
DtaP, 31, 175
DTP, 14, 31, 70
Dysbiosis, 11, 59, 132

E

Ear infections, 27, 32, 34, 46, 50
Eggs, 35, 91, 132, 133, 143
Electrolytes, 90, 144, 155
Elimination diet, 36, 96, 103, 139, 193
Environmental assault, 14
Environmental Factors, 19
Enzymes, 32, 35, 40, 45, 47, 49, 50, 54, 59, 82, 85, 86, 93, 99, 104, 105, 108, 116, 127, 139, 147, 173, 184
EPA, 83, 158
Epigenetics, 10, 13
Epsom salt, 122, 185
Ethylmercury, 24
Evidence of Harm, 208
Excitotoxins, 82, 117

F

Fabric softeners, 123
Failsafe diet, 153
Fallon, Sally, 140, 145, 207
Far Infrared Sauna, 164
Fat, animal, 76
Fat, dietary, 50, 129
Fat, oxidation, 130
Fat, saturated, 131
Faulty sulfation, 17, 21, 33, 45, 52, 77, 81, 90, 104, 105, 117, 141, 184
Feast without Yeast, 107
Feingold Diet, 96, 104, 105, 140, 153, 184, 207
Feingold, Dr. Ben, 17, 117
Fennel Seed, 93
Fermented foods, 95, 100, 101, 107, 147, 148, 149, 150, 151, 154, 155, 201, 207
Fermenting, soaking, 146, 149
Fluoride, 32, 91, 123, 161
Folic acid,, 74
Food sensitivities, 11, 30, 32, 33, 34, 35, 36, 55, 66, 85, 96, 97, 102, 103, 110, 138, 139, 152, 193
Formula, infant, 88, 140
Fragrance, 122, 123, 185

G

GAGs, 46, 50, 70
G-alpha protein, 14, 31, 49, 70, 71
Gas, 33, 85, 93, 96, 106, 123, 156, 172, 202
Gastrin, 46, 50, 51
Gelatin, 118, 145
genetic disorders, 68
Genetically Modified Organisms, 119
Genetics, 3, 13
GFCF, 95
Ginkgo Biloba, 93
Gliadinomorphins, 85
Gliotoxins, 33, 80

Glucuronic acid, 151
Glutamate, 82, 117, 118, 174
Glutamate, free, 145
Glutamine, 82, 157, 158, 161
Glutathione, 6, 11, 14, 37, 42, 43, 44, 48, 50, 53, 54, 71, 79, 80, 81, 92, 93, 94, 158, 161, 173
Gluten, 22, 30, 35, 36, 44, 48, 85, 95, 97, 98, 116, 118, 128, 136, 179, 180, 181, 206
Gluten-Free and Casein-Free Diet, 36, 86, 97, 98, 105, 107, 128, 135, 136, 152, 179
Glycerin, 118
Glycine, 81, 145, 161, 200
Glyconutrients, 89, 90, 158
Glycosaminoglycans, 46, 49
GMO, 119
GMOs, 119, 120
Gotu Kola, 93
Grass-fed, 132, 202
Great Smokies Diagnostic Lab, 66, 67, 68

H

Haley, 20, 52, 79
Haley, Boyd, 20, 21
HCl, 50, 51, 56, 67, 122, 123
Heavy metals, 26
Hemp, 84
Hemp seeds, 143
Herpes simplex virus, 60
Histamine, 79, 198, 200. *See*
Homocysteine, 40
Household Clean up, 122
Houston Nutraceuticals, 85, 179, 185, 208
Hyperactivity, 33, 35, 47, 80, 82, 85, 86, 96, 102, 104
Hyperammonemia,, 60
Hypothyroidism, 18, 55

I

IgA, 131
IgG, 46, 85, 91, 103, 138, 139
Immune function, 11
Immune System Support, 158
Infants, 52, 88, 140, 175, 176
Inflammation, 11, 30, 31, 35, 36, 44, 50, 51, 55, 58, 71, 78, 84, 85, 90, 92, 93, 95, 100, 106, 113, 116, 136, 138, 147, 159
Inositol, 74, 75
Ionic, 145
Iron, 143

J

James, 42, 214
Juicing, 145

K

Kefir, 88, 101, 149, 154
Ketogenic diet, 61
Kirby, David, 208
Kombu, 143, 144

kombucha, 149, 150, 151, 154, 155

L

Lactic Acid, 151
Lang, Michael, 33, 46, 49, 50, 71, 73, 77, 80, 81, 82, 90
Lard, 75
Lathe, Richard, 11, 58
Lead, 26, 79, 126, 200, 211
leafy greens, 76, 79, 105, 143
Leaky gut, 30, 32, 35, 36, 44, 71, 113
LEAP test, 66, 139, 198, 208
Lectin Lock and NAG, 92
Lectins, 147
Lettuce, 76
Ley, 88
Lipotropic nutrients, 161
Liver, 143
Low Oxalate Diet, 96, 106, 107, 153, 200, 201, 207
Lupus, 18

M

Magnesium, 55, 57, 61, 73, 77, 79, 88, 91, 98, 143, 144, 145, 147, 185
Malic Acid, 151
Manganese, 27, 211
McCandless, Jaquelyn, 60, 61, 64, 71, 72, 73, 74, 78, 79, 80, 82, 83, 84, 91, 205
Measles, 28, 29, 30, 32, 46, 49, 175
Medicinal Mushrooms, 89
Megson, Mary, 14, 31, 32, 70, 71
Melatonin, 59, 68, 91, 92, 132
Mercola, Dr., 99, 207
Mercury, 20, 21, 22, 26, 27, 28, 33, 44, 46, 47, 49, 52, 53, 72, 79, 83, 93, 113, 123, 162, 175
Mercury Toxicity, 19, 208
Mercury, effects of, 20
Mercury, elemental, 19
Mercury, inorganic, 19, 20, 24
Mercury, organic, 19
Methionine, 40, 43, 44, 50, 54, 91, 161, 184, 214
Methylation, 15, 16, 17, 21, 22, 33, 37, 40, 42, 44, 48, 59, 68, 91, 141, 153, 161. *See*
Methylation, DNA, 13
Methylmercury, 19, 23
Milk Thistle, 93
MMR, 29, 30, 175
MSG, 117, 118, 135, 181, 182, 196
MSM, 77, 185
MTHFR, 14
Multivitamin/mineral, 76
Myelination, 52

N

NAC, 77, 80, 91
Natural remedies, 157
Nettles, 143, 144
Neurodevelopment, 52
Neuroimmune, 11
Neurological disorder, 5

Neurological disorders, 17, 48, 49, 74, 105
Neurotoxin, 42, 46, 47
Neurotoxins, 27, 123
Nordic Naturals, 83
Nourishing Traditions, 140, 207
Nucleic Acids, 151
Nut milk. See
Nutrient-Dense Foods, 143
Nuts, 143, 144

O

Omega 3, 130
Omega 6, 130
Omega 9, 131
Omega-3, 83, 84, 143, 158, 217
Omega-6, 83, 84
Opiates, 11, 30, 35, 46, 48, 86, 116, 135
Owens, Susan, 45, 46, 47, 49, 52, 81, 200
Oxalates, 96, 106, 200, 201, 202, 203, 207
Oxalic Acid, 151
Oxytocin, 52

P

Pangborn, Jon, 175
Parasites, 50, 156
Pasteurization, 99
Pastured hens, 133
Pastured, hens, 143
Peptides, 35, 85
Perineuronal nets, 52
Pertussis, 11, 14, 31, 70, 212, 214
Pesticides, 27, 46, 60, 87, 119, 122, 142, 143, 212
Petroleum jelly and mineral oil, 124
Phase I, 48, 54, 161
Phenol intolerance, 47, 104, 105, 141
Phenolic, 47, 53, 96, 105, 108, 117, 122, 141, 161, 184
Phenolic exposure, 53
Phenols, 17, 47, 48, 53, 77, 95, 104, 105, 117, 118, 124, 135, 138, 140, 141, 161, 184, 185, 196
Phenolsulfotransferase (PST), 47
Phenylethylamine, 198
Phosphatidylcholine, 89
Phthalates, 124
Phytic acid, 147
Picky eaters/eating, 110
Pizzorno, 48, 49
Polymorphism, 13, 14, 15, 68
Poor eye contact, 20, 172
Potassium, 144
Pregnancy, 31, 140
Preservatives, 46, 103, 116, 117, 140, 196
Price, Weston A., 207
Probiotic, 86, 96, 127, 201
Probiotics, 34, 56, 86, 87, 88, 98, 107, 127, 155, 157, 158, 177, 213
Proinflammatory cytokines, 11
Proline, 145
Proteases, 85, 86
Protein, 50
Protein, dietary, 128, 132

PST, 45, 47, 117, 161
Psychological disorder, 5
Pycnogenol, 90, 160
Pyroluria, 62, 68, 78

R

Rapp, Dr. Doris, 35, 208
Raw Food Diet, 108
Raw milk, 55, 190
Rheumatoid arthritis, 18. *See* Arthritis
Rimland, Bernard, 73
RNA, 40
Rotation diet, 96, 102, 103, 104, 139, 148
Rubella, 31, 175

S

Salicylates, 47, 77, 105, 140, 161, 184, 207
Salt, 94, 145, 204
Salt, Himalayan crystal, 94, 145, 208
SAM, 40, 91
Sarsaparilla, 93
Sauerkraut, raw, 88, 91, 150, 154
Schisandra, 94
Seaweed, 143
Secretin, 50, 51
Seizures, 27, 60, 61, 104, 172, 184
Selenium, 24, 57, 64, 71, 79, 143, 158, 201
Serotonin, 132
Sleeping difficulties, 20
Soaking, 148
Sources of Exposure, 22
Soy, 35, 133
Specific Carbohydrate Diet (SCD), 60, 95, 98, 99, 100, 105, 118, 133, 149, 152, 192
Stock, meat, 144
Stoll, 83
Sugar, 35, 77, 79, 93, 95, 97, 98, 99, 103, 107, 118, 150, 151, 154
Sulfate, 17, 44, 45, 46, 47, 48, 49, 50, 51, 52, 90, 91, 104, 154, 173, 184, 185, 186
Sulfation, 17, 44, 45, 47, 48, 49, 50, 51, 52, 53, 67, 90, 104, 105, 117, 122, 124, 140, 141, 161, 184
Sulfotransferases, 45, 46, 49
Sweet potatoes, 143

T

T cell, 78, 81
Taurine, 35, 44, 56, 61, 64, 81, 82, 161
Teflon, 124
Th1, 27, 30, 44, 53, 55, 83, 159, 173
Th2, 44, 53, 55, 173
Thimerosal, 20, 22, 24
Thyroid, 14, 31, 32, 68, 159
Thyroid hormones, 14, 58
TMG, 40, 80
Toxic burdens, 162
Toxic load, 47, 119

Toxin, environmental, 27, 60, 61, 67, 87, 145, 161
Toxin, microbial, 28, 31
Toxin, yeast, 33, 36
Toxins, 22, 31, 33, 36, 37, 44, 46, 48, 49, 50, 51, 60, 71, 72, 80, 93, 122, 128, 151, 156, 164, 184
Trace ingredients, 179
Traditional foods, 128, 144, 147, 149, 207
Trans fats, 119
Transfer factor, 88
Transfer factors, 158
Tryptophan, 132
Type 1 diabetes, 18, 75
Tyramine, 198

U

Ulcerative colitis, 18, 29, 30, 100

V

Vaccinations, 26, 27, 28, 29, 46, 52, 175, 176, 208, 211
Vegetarian, 133
Vitamin A, 32, 64, 70, 158, 190, 215
Vitamin B12, 73
Vitamin B6, 72
Vitamin C, 64, 71, 72, 80, 143, 151, 158, 161, 175, 200, 201
Vitamin D, 75, 190
Vitamin E, 71, 72, 79, 80, 143, 158
Vitamin K, 76, 158, 201, 218

W

Wakefield, Dr. Andrew, 29, 30, 50, 217
Waring, Rosemary, 17, 45, 50, 90
Wecker, Dr. Lynn, 218
Weston A. Price Foundation, 190
Wheat, 30, 32, 33, 35, 66, 97, 103, 135, 179, 180, 181
Whole grains, 143

X

Xenobiotics, 173
Xylitol, 118

Y

Yasko, Amy, 82
Yeast, 27, 32, 33, 34, 35, 36, 48, 49, 50, 60, 66, 67, 80, 85, 89, 91, 95, 97, 99, 100, 113, 118, 149, 150, 151, 154, 155, 156, 159
Yeast diet, 107, 152
Yeast infections, 33
Yeast overgrowth, 33, 34, 133, 134, 149, 152

Z

Zinc, 5, 25, 27, 44, 56, 62, 64, 77, 78, 79, 132, 143, 158, 161

ABOUT THE AUTHOR

Julie Matthews is an internationally respected Certified Nutrition Consultant specializing in autism spectrum disorder. She is an expert in applying food, nutrition, and diet to aid digestive health and systemic healing. She has deep knowledge of biomedical approaches, sulfation, and the disordered chemistry of ASD. As an autism nutritionist, she provides sound diet and supplement intervention guidance backed by scientific research and applied clinical experience.

Julie studied nutrition at California state-certified Bauman College, where she investigated the connection between chemicals in foods and children's behavior. Initially curious about ADD/ADHD, she quickly focused on autism spectrum disorders after she met a father who'd recovered his children from autism through diet and nutrition. The father, a chemist, soon became a mentor to Julie and set her afire on a mission to inform and empower others. She also holds a Bachelor of Science from U.C. Davis in Agricultural and Managerial Economics. Julie is a member of the National Association of Nutrition Professionals and sits on the Scientific Advisory Board of *The Autism File* magazine. She has been a Defeat Autism Now! (DAN!) Practitioner since 2002.

Julie is an autism nutrition educator at the leading medical autism conferences including; Defeat Autism Now (DAN!), Autism One, Autism Society of America, National Autism Association, US Autism & Asperger's Association, Autism Today, and the Mindd Foundation. She is also a presenter for Nourishing Our Children, a non-profit campaign of the Weston A. Price Foundation's San Francisco Chapter. She hosts a radio show in San Francisco, called *Reality Sandwich*, which addresses varied health and autism healing topics, and on Autism One Radio called *Nourishing Hope*. She writes for, and serves on the scientific advisory board of, the Autism File magazine, and publishes varied online newsletters/blogs. Julie is the creator of "Cooking To Heal"— an autism nutrition and cooking class that teaches "how to" techiques for autism diet implementation.

Julie routinely collaborates with pediatricians, family physicians, nutritionists and researchers. Her passion is supporting parents and children from around the world during one-on-one consultations. She provides private group education for autism support groups and autism-focused education centers in the US and abroad. Julie has a private autism nutrition practice in San Francisco, California, where she resides with her husband and daughter. She can be reached at NourishingHope.com.

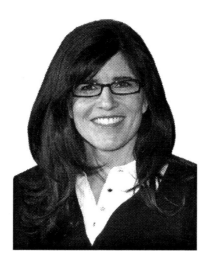

Independent Publisher Book Awards 2009

13TH ANNUAL AWARDS

Outstanding Book of the Year - Gold Medal Winner
"Most Progressive Health Book"

Nourishing Hope for Autism:
Nutrition Intervention for Healing Our Children

by Julie Matthews

Healthful Living Media

Sponsored by Jenkins Group Inc. & *IndependentPublisher.com*

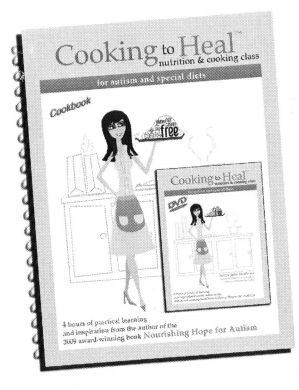
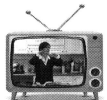
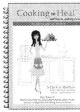
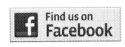

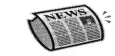